SECOND EDITION

AMERICAN CANCER SOCIETY

COMPLETE GUIDE TO

Family Caregiving

SECOND EDITION

AMERICAN CANCER SOCIETY

COMPLETE GUIDE TO

Family
Caregiving

The Essential Guide to Cancer Caregiving at Home

EDITED BY

Julia A. Bucher, RN, PhD
Peter S. Houts, PhD
Terri Ades, DNP, FNP-BC, AOCN

Published by the American Cancer Society/Health Promotions
250 Williams Street NW, Atlanta, Georgia 30303-1002 USA

Printed in the United States of America

Design and composition: LaShae V. Ortiz, New York, NY
Copy editing and indexing: Beth Allen, Houston, TX

5 4 3 2 1   11 12 13 14 15

Library of Congress Cataloging-in-Publication Data
American Cancer Society complete guide to family caregiving : the essential guide to cancer caregiving at home. —2nd ed. / edited by Julia A. Bucher, Peter S. Houts, and Terri Ades.
    p. cm.
    Rev. ed. of: Caregiving. Rev. ed. 2003.
    Includes bibliographical references and index.
    ISBN-13: 978-0-944235-00-3 (pbk. : alk. paper)
    ISBN-10: 0-944235-00-X (pbk. : alk. paper)
1. Cancer—Palliative treatment. 2. Cancer—Patients—Home care. 3. Caregivers. I. Bucher, Julia A. II. Houts, Peter S. III. Ades, Terri B. IV. American Cancer Society. V. Caregiving. VI. Title: Complete guide to family caregiving.
    RC271.P33C37 2011
    649.8—dc22   2010015968

AMERICAN CANCER SOCIETY
Managing Director, Content: Chuck Westbrook
Director, Book Publishing: Len Boswell
Managing Editor, Books: Rebecca Teaff, MA
Editor, Books: Jill Russell
Book Publishing Coordinator: Vanika Jordan, MSPub
Editorial Assistant, Books: Amy Rovere

For more information about cancer, contact your American Cancer Society at **800-227-2345** or **cancer.org**.

Quantity discounts on bulk purchases of this book are available. Book excerpts can also be created to fit specific needs. For information, please contact your American Cancer Society, Health Promotions Publishing, 250 Williams Street NW, Atlanta, Georgia 30303-1002, or send an e-mail to **trade.sales@cancer.org**.

A NOTE TO THE READER

The information in this book is not official policy of the American Cancer Society and is not intended as medical advice to replace the expertise and judgment of your cancer care team. It is intended to help you and your family make informed decisions, together with your doctor.

For more information about cancer, contact your American Cancer Society at **800-227-2345** or **cancer.org**.

CONTENTS

ACKNOWLEDGMENTS

Many people contributed to the development of this book. They include physicians, nurses, psychologists, and social workers, as well as people with cancer and their family and friends. Several individuals have been especially generous in contributing their time and expertise across the years and, as a result, have had a substantial influence on the development and growth of this book. For this revised second edition, we would like to thank the following contributors: Margaret Crowley, MSN, CRNP, APRN-BC; Cara Granda-Cameron, MSN, CRNP; Brigitte Haagen, DNSc; and Patricia Siegrist. In addition, we acknowledge the administrative support provided by the Department of Nursing, York College of Pennsylvania.

For previous editions of this book, we are deeply indebted to Regena Tripp, RN, OCN; David Houts; Charles Schreiber; Bruce Nicholson, MD; George Simms, MD; and the Cancer Prevention and Control unit of the Pennsylvania Department of Health. We also express our appreciation to the following people for their support and suggestions during this project: John Stryker, MD; Frank Davidoff, MD, FACP; Thomas Feagin, MD, FACP; Charles Lewis, MD, FACP; Nick Leasure, MD; David Hufford, PhD; Steven Hulse, MEd; Judy Lyter, RN; Catherine Kleese, RN, OCN; Mary Jo Templin, RN; Janice Mills, RN, MS; Bonnie Bixler, MEd; and Julia Yost.

Much of the information in this book was based on content from the first edition, which was created with the assistance of the contributors and reviewers below.

Reviewers, First Edition

Diane Blum, ACSW

Marjorie Cassel

Mary Ann Cegielsky, RN, MSN, OCN

Deborah Clark, RN, BSN

Margaret Davitt, RN, MSN

Diane Erdos, RN, MSN

Shirley Faddis, MSN, OCN

Timothy Freer

Sandra Frey, RN, OCN

Phyllis Hall, MSW

Edward Henry

Bonnie Koch, RN, OCN

Kenneth Kohler

Mary Lander, RN

Carolyn Messner, ACSW

Linda Mogul, MSW

Bruce Nicholson, MD

Sharon Olson, RN, MSN

Carol Ann Peters, RN, MSN

Harold Piety

Eric Pfeiffer, MS

James B. Ray, PharmD

Kathleen Rine, RN, MSN

Barbara Robinawitz, PhD

Susan A. Rokita, RN, MSN

Irena Rusenas, MS

Lori Sandohl, RN, DSN, CW, OCN

Marion Sattazahn

William Sattazahn, Jr.

Marion Spangler

Nancy Toth, RN

Barbara Van Horn

Katherine Yoder, RN, OCN

Renee Atchison Ziegler

Contributors, First Edition

Carole A. Bean
Georgia Brown, RN
Elise M. Givant, RN, OCN
Harold A. Harvey, MD
Joan F. Hermann, LSW
Kathy B. Kambic, RN, OCN
Mary Lander, RN
Allan Lipton, MD
Matthew J. Loscalzo, MSW
Arthur M. Nezu, PhD

Christine M. Nezu, PhD
Bruce Nicholson, MD
Carol Nolt, MSW
Eric Pfeiffer, MS
Dale B. Schelzel, RN, OCN
Mary A. Simmonds, MD
Sandra J. Spoljaric, RN, OCN
Glenda M. Trumpower, MSW
James R. Zabora, MSW, ScD

Administrative Support, First Edition

Departments of Behavioral Science and Medicine, Penn State University College of Medicine
Department of Clinical and Health Psychology, School of Health Professionals, Allegheny
     University of the Health Sciences
Department of Nursing, Bloomsburg University of Pennsylvania
Johns Hopkins Oncology Center

American Cancer Society

INTRODUCTION

When a person receives a cancer diagnosis, life changes. But life also changes for the caregiver who helps that person get through the cancer experience. The caregiver— whether it be a spouse, partner, adult child, or friend—also participates in the experience, filling a role that is crucial to the physical and emotional well-being of the person with cancer.

Changes in health care have led to an increase in the involvement of family and friends in the day-to-day home care of the person with cancer. Today, cancer treatment is often administered on an outpatient basis instead of in the hospital. Even when treatments are done in the hospital, the patient typically spends less time there than in the past. With such changes, the role of primary caregiver becomes multifaceted—ranging from home health care aide to companion.

The caregiver may take on responsibilities that, just a short time ago, were reserved for trained health care professionals. Caregivers and patients themselves have the responsibility of monitoring medications, managing side effects, and reporting conditions or situations that require professional intervention. The caregiver may help feed, dress, and bathe the person with cancer, as well as arrange schedules, manage insurance issues, and provide transportation. Caregivers serve as legal assistants, financial managers, and housekeepers. They often have to take over the duties the person with cancer once performed, while continuing to meet other family members' needs. In addition, a caregiver can have an enormous influence on how the person with cancer deals with his or her illness. The caregiver's encouragement can help the person with cancer stick with a demanding treatment plan and take other steps that are necessary to get well, such as eating nutritious meals and getting enough rest.

Cancer care is more complex today than ever before. Scientific and technical advances in the early detection, diagnosis, and treatment of cancer have increased the chances of extending life and have even increased the chances of cure for many types of cancer. Treatment plans often combine surgery, radiation therapy, chemotherapy, and other therapies. Frequent tests are required to monitor the effects of treatment. Cancer treatments often continue for months.

After treatment ends, cancer recurrence may force treatments to resume. Therefore, people with cancer, their families, and all caregivers must be prepared to cope with a wide range of physical, emotional, and social consequences of the disease and treatments, often for extended periods.

The *American Cancer Society Complete Guide to Family Caregiving, Second Edition* provides guidance to caregivers and people with cancer for coping with the challenges of illness and treatment. This book was written by cancer care professionals with many years of experience, with input from home caregivers and people with cancer. This book supplies the information needed to manage care, prepare for cancer treatment and potential side effects, and prevent problems rather than just respond to crises. This book also can help patients and caregivers work more cooperatively with health care professionals.

Caring for someone with cancer can be fulfilling, but it can also be demanding and stressful. There is almost always too much for just one person to do. Asking for help or allowing others to help can relieve some of the pressures of caregiving and, in turn, allow caregivers to also take care of themselves.

How to Use This Book

This book consists of five sections: Managing Care, Emotional Responses to Cancer and Cancer Treatment, Physical Side Effects of Cancer and Cancer Treatment, Living with Longer-Term Side Effects of Cancer Treatment, and Transitioning from Curing to Caring, in addition to two appendices, a resource guide, and a glossary.

The first section summarizes some of the basics of caregiving, such as how to approach the challenges of caregiving, grasping the complexities of the caregiver role, and helping to prepare children in the person's life for the changes that come with cancer and its treatment. This section also deals with the practical issues of caregiving, including coordinating care, getting help from community resources, obtaining information from medical staff, and managing the financial aspects of treatment.

The three subsequent sections—Emotional Responses to Cancer and Cancer Treatment, Physical Side Effects of Cancer and Cancer Treatment, and Living with Longer-Term Side Effects of Cancer Treatment—cover situations or conditions that may occur during cancer care and explore how the caregiver can help.

The final section—Transitioning from Curing to Caring—deals with the situations caregivers face when the focus is no longer on curing the person, but on caring for them. This section will not be appropriate for everyone reading this book. But for caregivers and patients who are facing the end of a loved one's life, this can be a stressful and difficult time. This section provides guidance for the person with cancer as well as the caregiver and family.

Appendix A summarizes the major types of cancer treatment and clinical trials. It explains the different treatments, why and when they are used, and the effects they can have on people receiving the treatments. Appendix B summarizes food safety guidelines for people undergoing cancer treatment. The resource guide provides a listing of organizations, programs, and services for those affected by cancer. The glossary offers readers a guide to common terms for quick reference.

When to Read the Chapters

We recommend reading as much as you can before you attempt to deal with any problems. Reading the chapters early allows you to develop plans that you can refine as you gain experience. Having plans will also give you a sense of confidence and purpose that can help you cope with the stresses of caregiving. By reading a chapter before problems develop, you will be able to recognize them early, take action before they become severe, and even prevent some problems from happening.

Reread chapters when situations or conditions persist. These chapters contain many strategies for dealing with caregiving situations or conditions. It can be hard to remember them all. Reread chapters when a problem occurs or persists to be sure you are doing everything you can.

Encourage the person with cancer to read relevant chapters. This book isn't just for caregivers. The person with cancer needs to understand the care plans and participate in carrying them out if they are to be successful. People with cancer are often their own caregivers, especially if they live alone or if family and friends rely on them for instructions. If you have cancer and are reading this book, we suggest you think of yourself as your own caregiver.

Using Problem Solving in Caregiving

Caregivers must, on some level, be problem solvers. In one way or another, you have been solving problems throughout your life. The only difference now is that many of the challenges that come with cancer are new to you and to the person for whom you are caring. This book will help both of you through these new challenges.

In many ways, your caregiving experience will be a process of confronting challenges and helping your loved one deal with these challenges. This book advocates an approach to the problem solving of caregiving that we call "COPE." The term COPE stands for **Creativity**, **Optimism**, **Planning**, and **Expert information**. Using the COPE ideas in problem solving will help make the tasks of caregiving more manageable, can help you feel a sense of accomplishment in your work as a caregiver, and—most important—will enable you to give the best possible care.

Not all of the ideas in this chapter will apply to every situation or problem. But it can be easy to feel stuck or overwhelmed when dealing with a tough problem or condition. The COPE acronym is a reminder to help you think in a different way and help you remember what to do when you feel stuck. Here is how to use each of the COPE ideas.

"C" is for Creativity

Most plans, no matter how well thought out, will run into obstacles or roadblocks. When you run into obstacles, try to see the problem as a challenge to your creativity. Begin thinking creatively about overcoming challenges that could prevent you from reaching your goal. There are many ways to be creative:

1. **Talk to someone about the problem or imagine what another person would do about the problem.** Explaining a problem to someone else helps you see it more clearly. You can also imagine that you are talking to someone, which can help you see the problem

more clearly without another person actually being there. Other people also may think of ideas that you would not have thought of alone.

2. **Improve on an idea that worked to some extent.** Too often we discard ideas that had some positive effect because they weren't completely successful. If an idea was partly successful, try thinking about what was good about that idea, and use that as a basis for a new one.

3. **Try a smaller goal.** Sometimes we become disappointed because we expect change to happen too fast. We think we are not successful when, in reality, we are making progress. A creative solution may be to scale down what you hope to accomplish so that it matches what you can accomplish. In other words, "If at first you don't succeed, try a smaller goal."

4. **Brainstorm.**
   Make a list of ideas that might be useful. Make your list as long as possible, and do not censor yourself. Any ideas you have, no matter how strange or silly, should be included on the list.
   Combine good ideas into better ideas. When you have finished your list, go over it and try to combine good ideas to make even better ideas.
   Choose ideas most likely to be successful. Finally, go over your list again with a critical eye and choose the ideas that you think have the best chance of being successful.

"O" is for Optimism

One of the most important things you can do to help the person you are caring for is to remain optimistic. That doesn't mean sugarcoating or being unrealistic. Optimism can mean remembering to encourage your loved one or remind him or her of progress. People who are dealing with the stress of cancer and cancer treatments need encouragement and may need help noticing the good things that are happening. At the same time, it is important to be realistic about the seriousness of their problems so that they do not feel that their problems are being ignored. Here are some ways to make optimism part of your caregiving experience:

1. **Set reasonable goals.** The day-to-day issues of coping with cancer can be overwhelming for both patient and caregiver. One of the best ways to remain optimistic in the face of overwhelming circumstances is to break situations into manageable pieces and set reasonable goals. If goals are reasonable, you have a better chance of succeeding, which helps in keeping a positive attitude. Learning to resolve big issues in small steps is an important part of good caregiving.

2. **Expect to succeed.** If you think that you stand a good chance of success, you will do your best. If you become discouraged and negative, ask for help from someone who has a positive attitude and who is a good problem solver. This could be a friend, family member, or health care professional.

3. **Take breaks from caregiving.** Caregiving can be draining. Take breaks to do things that you enjoy. Taking breaks will help you maintain a positive outlook, even when you feel stressed. Read the chapter "Being an Effective Caregiver" (beginning on page 5) for ideas and guidance on dealing with your feelings as a caregiver. In addition, the chapters "Anxiety" (pages 71–78) and "Depression" (pages 79–90) can apply as much to the caregiver as they do to the person with cancer. These chapters can help you to cope with your situation and better face the challenges that come with caregiving.

4. **Accept that problems are inevitable.** Problems are part of life, and having them when you are taking care of someone is normal and common. Ask yourself, "How have my problems changed since I became a caregiver?" Many problems will be the same as before the cancer experience, others will be worse, but some problems will be better. For example, maybe a frustrating repair problem with your house has been resolved, or maybe a minor work irritation has blown over.

5. **Realize that you are already an effective problem solver.** Solving the problems that come with caregiving takes training and practice. But you have a head start—you have been dealing with problems all of your life, whether at home, at work, with friends, or with family. You are capable of solving caregiving problems, too.

6. **Try different ways of staying optimistic.**

   Use positive self-talk. Try to frame situations in a positive light. If you are feeling tired and overwhelmed, you might say to yourself, "I'm always tired and can never get to the things I need to get done." This "self-message" will make you feel depressed. If instead you say to yourself, "I am feeling tired now, but I'm looking forward to taking time tomorrow to do some things I want to do," you will have made a promise to yourself that will help you feel positive and hopeful.

   Control negative self-talk. Avoid using words like "should" or "ought" and replace them with "hope" and "try." Instead of saying, "I **should** invite my friends to visit," say, "I will **try** to invite my friends to visit."

   Challenge your own irrational beliefs and overgeneralizations. If you think, "I'm a failure," challenge that thought. Say to yourself, "No, that's wrong. I have been successful, and here is a time when I was a success." Then remind yourself of a success. Question words such as *disaster* and *hopeless*, and think carefully about what really happened.

   Use positive self-statements, such as "I **can** solve this problem," "I **can** cope with this," "I **can** reduce my fears," or "It's **normal** to feel upset in this situation."

   Use your feelings as cues or signals. Feelings tell you that a problem needs to be solved. Negative feelings may be a sign that a problem is present. Use your negative feelings to help you begin your problem-solving efforts.

If you are feeling anxious or down, read the chapter on depression in this book. The chapter on depression (beginning on page 79) can help you manage negative feelings. It will also help you evaluate the severity of symptoms, determine whether professional help is needed, and find help if necessary.

"P" is for Planning

Planning is essential to dealing with the challenges of caregiving. In the case of complex challenges, this can mean actually writing down a plan. It may just mean approaching problems in an orderly way. Follow these guidelines when developing your caregiving plans:

1. **Start by getting the facts.** You need to know the facts about your situation in order to solve a problem It helps to think of yourself as a detective or investigative reporter. Do not guess or assume. Separate what might be true from what you know to be true. Your job is to determine, with as much certainty as possible, the facts about the problem and to match those facts with information in this book about what can be done about the problem. For example, perhaps the person seems confused and you are not sure why. Begin with what you know and consult the chapter "Confusion and Seizures," beginning on page 209.

2. **Break down the problem into clear, specific details and use objective words.** Instead of saying, "I'm upset because nothing happens the way I want it to," try, "I feel upset because I don't have the time to visit my friend." By stating your problem precisely, other people can understand exactly what you mean, and you give yourself a clear goal to work toward (in this case, visiting your friend).

3. **Separate facts from impressions and assumptions.** For example, think about the difference between the statement, "She doesn't like me anymore," and, "When I passed her in the hall, she didn't notice me." The second way of stating the problem does not make assumptions about the other person's thoughts or motivations. It states the facts and leaves open the possibility that there was another reason the person did not notice you.

4. **Identify exactly what makes the condition or situation a problem.** It is not productive to panic and say, "He's getting worse." Instead, identify exactly what the problem is. For example, "He feels warm, and I wonder if a fever might be starting." The first statement is too general, but the second statement points to an action: take his temperature and read the chapter "Fever and Infections" to decide whether you should call a doctor.

5. **Develop your plan.** Think about what you and other people need to do to reach your goal. Involve the person you are caring for as much as possible in developing and carrying out the plan. It should be his or her plan as well as yours. If others are involved, think

about how you will work with them. If professional help is needed, that should be your first priority. Instructions from the person's doctor and the sections on when to get professional help in chapters 1–26 will give you guidance.

6. **Carry out, evaluate, and adjust your plan.**

   Review the sections at the end of each chapter on carrying out and adjusting your plan. These sections will offer suggestions on how to organize your plans. They also recommend things to do if your plan is not working.

   Set deadlines to be sure things will get done. Setting deadlines can help keep you on track and ensure that important tasks get done.

   Keep a record or diary of what you did and the results. Keeping a record will help you see what was successful and will give you ideas for dealing with similar problems in the future. A record will also help you when you're discussing problems with medical staff.

   If your plan isn't working, reevaluate. Review what you have done and the results. Revise your plan and keep trying.

"E" is for Expert Information

If you have questions or concerns about your loved one's treatment or any other aspect of his or her care, it is important that you rely on trustworthy and reliable sources of information. Follow these guidelines to obtain expert information:

1. **Seek out reliable resources.** You can always ask members of the health care team for information and recommendations. The resource guide at the end of this book lists established organizations that can provide reliable information about cancer and its treatment. There are also many books and Web sites available that give information and guidance. Be wary, however, of any source promoting a specific treatment or product or making promises that sound too good to be true. Information about many topics related to cancer and its treatment is available by calling your American Cancer Society at **800-227-2345** or visiting its Web site, **cancer.org**.

2. **Consider whether professional help is needed.** In each of the chapters discussing an emotional or physical condition the person with cancer might experience, there is a section on "When to Get Professional Help." These sections outline the situations or circumstances in which a health care provider should be called.

3. **Identify what you can do.** If professional help is not needed (or if that help has already been given), there are still things you can do to manage the problem on your own. Refer to the sections "What You Can Do" in chapters 1–26. These list what other people have found helpful in managing caregiving problems. You can also get ideas from family, friends, support groups, and from community service agencies and hospital staff.

Additional information, resources, and support for caregivers and people with cancer are available through your local office of the American Cancer Society, on the Web at **cancer.org**, or by calling **800-227-2345**, any time, day or night.

Part I

Managing Care

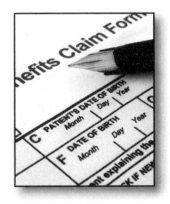

TAKING CARE OF SOMEONE WITH CANCER CAN BE A DAUNTING TASK. This section explores some essential ideas to help you be the best caregiver possible. Chapter 1, "Being an Effective Caregiver," examines the many roles the family caregiver must play and discusses the importance of taking care of yourself during this challenging time. Chapter 2, "Helping Children Understand," explores ways to help children, from toddlers through adolescents, whose lives have been affected by the cancer diagnosis. Chapters 3 through 6 focus on coordinating care from one treatment setting to another, getting help from community agencies, getting information from medical professionals, and managing the financial aspects of cancer and cancer treatment.

These guidelines are appropriate to most situations, but every situation has its unique issues. Always follow your health care team's instructions. Encourage the person with cancer to read this information, and then you can work together as a team.

For more information on any of the topics discussed in this section, contact your American Cancer Society at **800-227-2345** or visit the Web site at **cancer.org**.

CHAPTER ONE

Being an Effective Caregiver

Caregivers have an important and unique role to play in helping a person with cancer through his or her cancer experience. Caring for someone with cancer can be demanding and stressful. You may feel overwhelmed and depleted at times. You will need to ask for help sometimes.

Caregiving can also be fulfilling. Try not to forget the positive parts of caregiving. Some caregivers see taking care of someone with cancer as their lifework. Many feel that family caregiving has enriched their lives. Others see it as a challenge and want to do the best job they can. Some see caregiving as a way of showing appreciation for the love and care they themselves have received. Others see caregiving as spiritually enriching.

Caring for a person with cancer at home can give you a sense of satisfaction and confidence. It can reveal inner strengths you did not realize you had. It can draw families together and can help people feel closer to the person who needs care.

Caregiving can also open doors to new friends and relationships through talking to other people who have faced the same problems. These relationships could include people from a support group, health professionals who show understanding and concern, and family members who have grown distant but who are drawn together because of this difficult situation.

When to Get Professional Help

Ask for help from health care professionals, social workers, a member of the clergy, or other professionals if any of the following conditions exist:

- ***You are not able to carry out your caregiving responsibilities, and the needs of the person with cancer are not being met.*** Health care professionals, social workers, and clergy can help you get the help you need so the person with cancer gets needed help and services.

- **You are experiencing severe anxiety or depression.** It is normal to feel upset and stressed when caring for someone with cancer. Read the chapters on anxiety and depression for a list of symptoms that indicate whether you need professional help to cope. Getting professional help for anxiety or depression is just like getting help for physical problems. It is not a sign of weakness and is not a reason to be embarrassed. It means that you are wise and even courageous. Professionals such as social workers, counselors, clergy, psychologists, and psychiatrists are skilled and experienced in helping people who are facing difficult challenges. Your family doctor also can be helpful in assessing your symptoms and recommending a professional to help you.

- **Communication between you and the person with cancer has broken down or has become painful or difficult.** The stresses that come with cancer—physical, psychological, financial, and emotional—can interfere with your ability to communicate with the person for whom you are caring. Get professional help if anxiety and stress levels have risen to a level that prevents you from talking openly with the person about important issues.

- **Your relationship with the person with cancer is clouded by a history of abuse or addiction.** If you have experienced verbal, mental, physical, or sexual abuse from the person for whom you are caring, you are likely to have serious problems in caregiving. You may already have strong and deep-seated feelings, usually built up over many years. These feelings may come from past problems with alcohol or drug addiction that hurt family relationships or friendships. A history of abuse calls for professional help from the start of caregiving.

What You Can Do

This chapter outlines four important goals to keep in mind in your caregiving:

- **Work as a team** with the person with cancer and with health professionals, family, and friends.
- **Communicate with the person with cancer** in order to involve him or her as much as possible.
- **Be an advocate** for the person with cancer to be sure that he or she gets the information and services that are needed.
- **Take care of your own needs** so that you have the emotional and physical strength to be a helpful and effective caregiver.

Start using the ideas in this chapter now. Don't wait until you feel overwhelmed. It is easier to develop good caregiving habits and attitudes early on before problems get out of hand. Set reasonable goals for yourself. It takes time and experience to improve your caregiving skills. Be patient with yourself.

Every week or so, take time to think about how you are doing as a caregiver. Think back over your experiences, and try to pay attention to how much you have learned and how you have improved. Reread this chapter periodically to see whether there are ideas here that can be of help.

Work as a Team

In cancer care, the person with cancer, health care professionals, and family members and friends are all members of the care team. The family caregiver is a team player—working with the person with cancer, with other family and friends, and with health care staff to solve problems.

⟼ Include the person with cancer.

The person with cancer is central to the team. His or her participation in care and involvement in all problem-solving discussions is critical and requires the person's cooperation and agreement.

⟼ Include health care professionals.

Health care professionals are also key members of the team. Working with and communicating with health care professionals will ensure that the care given at home is consistent with the best medical and home care practices.

⟼ Involve family and friends.

Family members and friends who share in caregiving are also important team members. In addition to helping in practical ways, family members and friends can give encouragement and emotional support. They also can share their experiences and knowledge from dealing with similar problems in their lives.

Communicate with the Person with Cancer

Working well and communicating clearly with the person with cancer is your most important job. It can also be the most challenging. The person for whom you are caring is dealing with the physical effects of the disease and treatments as well as the psychological and social challenges of living with cancer. These problems may make it difficult for him or her to participate in making decisions or plans. Nonetheless, your job is to involve him or her as much as possible in making decisions and carrying out plans.

➡ **Create a climate that encourages sharing feelings and supports the person's efforts to share.**

Talk about important or sensitive topics in a time and place that's calm and favorable to open communication—not in the midst of a crisis or an argument. If your time for talking about important issues in your family is around the dinner table, that's the time and place to do it. Think about when and where you have had important and constructive talks in the past. Strive to recreate that setting.

➡ **Communicate your availability.**

One of the most important messages you can communicate is that you are available and willing to listen and talk when the person wants to discuss issues. However, leave the timing up to him or her. As much as possible, the person with cancer should make decisions on what feelings to share and when, how, and with whom to share them. By not pressing the issue, you allow the person to retain control over part of his or her life at a time when many circumstances and decisions are beyond his or her control.

➡ **Understand that men and women often communicate in different ways, and make allowances for those differences.**

In our society, women are sometimes encouraged or taught to express their feelings more openly than men. If you are a man caring for a woman, be aware when she shares her feelings. You may find yourself giving advice when she just wants someone to listen and be understanding. On the other hand, if you are a woman caring for a man, be aware that he may express his feelings differently from how you might. Pay special attention when he talks about things that are important to him. It may be helpful to openly discuss differences in how men and women express their feelings and share how you would like to be supported. Also, remember that we spend our lifetimes developing communication styles, and they won't change overnight.

➡ **Be realistic and flexible about the person's communication preferences.**

People with cancer may want or need to share and discuss many things, but they may not want to share them all with just one person. Let the person talk about whatever he or she wants with whomever he or she wants. It's okay if the person isn't telling you everything, as long as he or she is telling somebody.

➡ **Remember that sharing doesn't always mean talking.**

The person with cancer may feel more comfortable writing about his or her feelings or expressing them through an activity. He or she may express feelings in other nonverbal ways, such as by making gestures or expressions, touching, or just asking that you be present. Sharing someone's silence can be a wonderful experience and a privilege. Similarly, sometimes the person with cancer may need to be alone. As a caregiver, try to respect the person's right to be alone.

⦀➡ Remember that you don't have to agree.

Two people are not always at the same place about important issues at the same time. There is no simple answer to many problems—especially problems that last a long time.

⦀➡ Explain your needs openly.

You, the caregiver, will also have needs. Sometimes you may need to ask the person with cancer to do something to make your life easier or make your caregiving responsibilities easier. Keep in mind that conflict resolution does not always mean everybody is happy. On some issues, compromise might be appropriate. On other issues, you may have to give in or ask the other person to give in.

⦀➡ Suggest a trial run or time limit.

If you want the person with cancer to try something (such as a new bed or a new medicine schedule) and he or she is resisting, ask to try it for a limited time, such as a week, and then evaluate the change. This approach avoids making the person feel locked into a decision. For example, if you want the person with cancer to ring a bell to call for help when in bed and he or she thinks it is unnecessary, ask the person to try your idea for a few days. Then you can talk about how it worked and whether it should continue.

⦀➡ Choose your battles carefully.

Ask yourself, "What's really important here? Am I being stubborn because I need to win an argument?" You can save energy by skipping minor conflicts and using your energy and influence on issues that really count. For example, you might be willing to press the issue when it comes to the person getting enough rest or taking important medications. If not all of the person's food choices are as healthy as you'd like, however, this might be an area where you choose not to argue.

⦀➡ Let the person with cancer continue to make decisions about his or her life.

Taking away a person's ability to make decisions can undermine his or her feelings of control. For example, an adult child living far from an ill parent might want to move the parent into a nursing home so that someone will be there to help the person if there are any problems. Although this move might make the adult child feel better, it may not be what the parent wants. If the person with cancer understands the consequences of his or her decision (for example, in the case of the parent, that no one may be around to help if he or she falls), he or she has the right to make that decision.

▥➔ **Help the person cope with the diagnosis and live as normal a life as possible.**
Living as normal a life as possible can be a good way to cope with cancer. By helping the person with cancer maintain normal routines, you can minimize the disruptions caused by cancer and its treatment. However, some people try to deal with the emotional stress of a cancer diagnosis by pretending that it's not happening. This could be harmful if the person does things that make the illness worse, such as avoiding medical treatment, canceling visits to the doctor, or pursuing activities that could be harmful. It is important to have realistic expectations about activity levels while undergoing treatment and to avoid activities that could be harmful.

Be an Advocate

An advocate talks to the person with cancer about his or her needs and helps make sure those needs are met. As an advocate, you can help the person to help him or herself, or you can step in for the person, with permission, and speak up for his or her needs. An advocate is someone that the person with cancer looks to for assistance and advice. It is a very special role.

One of the ways that caregivers can help is to serve as an advocate for the person with cancer. In order to be an effective advocate in the health care system, the caregiver must strive to understand the needs of the person with cancer and to help make sure those needs are met.

▥➔ **Ask questions.**
Asking questions is the best way to make sure that you understand what will happen during treatment. Help the person with cancer prepare a written list of questions before appointments, procedures, and treatments. Offer to take notes during appointments so the person with cancer can concentrate on listening. If the person with cancer does not feel comfortable asking specific questions because of nervousness or embarrassment, the caregiver can help ask these difficult questions and record the answers.

Make sure you understand the goal of any test, procedure, or treatment, as well as what can be expected afterwards, including side effects and recovery times. Make sure you understand instructions for any at-home care necessary after procedures or treatments. Ask whether there are educational materials available about the condition, procedure, or treatment beforehand—or go out and do some research. The more information you have, the better prepared you can be.

▥➔ **Keep detailed health records.**
Caregivers can also help the person with cancer maintain a personal health record. This record should include a detailed summary of the person's health history along with copies of records kept by the person's health care team and any other treatment providers and insurers. Don't hesitate to ask for copies of these records; the patient has a right to his or her information. The person with cancer will have to name you as an approved recipient of these private medical records

for them to be released directly to you. Otherwise it will be necessary for the person with cancer to place the request. This record should be kept up-to-date either on a computer or stored in a binder for easy reference. Make sure to include medications, dosages, and dates of treatment along with any allergies or reactions to medications. Also include any vitamins, dietary supplements, or over-the-counter medications taken by the person with cancer. Have a list of the person's health care providers and their contact information available in the event there are questions about treatment records.

Make sure friends, family members, and other caregivers know the location of this personal health information. It may not always be easy for the person with cancer to recall this history from memory, especially in the event of an emergency. Having a personal health record available can make sure that important information is not overlooked when the person needs medical care.

⯈ Help the person manage financial issues.

Depending on the situation and your relationship to the person, you may need to assist with the management of the household finances and issues related to payment for cancer treatment. The finances of paying for cancer treatment can be complex, and you may need to help the person with keeping records and organization of the family's finances. See chapter 6 for more information.

⯈ Express concerns.

It is essential that you speak up if you have any concerns about the person's care. Know your rights. If you are not satisfied with the care the person with cancer receives, you have the right to speak up. First, talk to the doctor or nurse. You can also speak with a social worker at the hospital or treatment center to help resolve any problems. If these problems are not resolved to your satisfaction, you have the right to seek treatment from another provider.

Take Care of Your Own Needs

Caregivers also need to take care of themselves. Helping someone who is going through cancer and its treatment can be difficult and stressful. As a caregiver, the more you care for your own needs for sleep, rest, food, friendships, enjoyment, and relaxation, the better you will be able to help the person for whom you are caring. Taking time for yourself and remembering to notice the good things still happening in both of your lives will help you to be a better caregiver.

Caregivers need to be at their best to do the best job of caregiving. Be aware of your own needs as well as those of the person you are helping. Set limits on what you can reasonably expect of yourself. Take time off to care for yourself and your own needs. Ask for help before stress builds up.

⟫ **Take time for positive experiences.**

There are many types of positive experiences that can promote good mental health. Make sure you schedule positive experiences for yourself.

- *Pursue enjoyable activities with other people.*
  Have lunch with a friend, attend a support group meeting, or enjoy an activity with someone you love.
- *Engage in activities that impart a sense of accomplishment.*
  Cook a special meal, exercise, or finish a scrapbook.
- *Pursue activities that just promote feeling good or relaxing.*
  Watch a funny movie, play with a pet, or take a walk.

Plan these activities regularly, and, when you are away from caregiving, try to be completely away from it. You can recharge your batteries, so to speak, by being involved and absorbed in something besides caregiving. It may be beneficial to talk to a friend about the challenges you are facing and how caregiving is affecting you.

Pay attention to positive experiences in your everyday life and routines. Make an effort to notice and talk about pleasant experiences as they happen during the day. Do a crossword puzzle or take time to read the morning paper or a magazine. Set aside time during the day, such as during a meal, when you and the person with cancer do not discuss the illness.

⟫ **Find ways to deal with strong feelings.**

It is natural to have strong feelings when taking care of someone with a serious illness like cancer. The following is a list of strong feelings that caregivers can have and strategies for dealing with them if they become severe.

Feeling overwhelmed

Sometimes problems from caregiving and from other parts of your life build up to the point where you feel overwhelmed. Consider these suggestions if you are feeling overwhelmed:

- *Try not to make important decisions when upset.*
  Sometimes you have to make decisions immediately, but often you don't. Ask the doctor, nurse, or social worker how long you have before a particular decision has to be made.
- *Take time to sort things out.*
  It is important to take some time to let your thinking become clear again. Different people need different amounts of time to find clarity. Give yourself enough time to become more emotionally stable so that you can make plans and decisions with a clear mind and a peaceful spirit.

- **Break down problems into smaller problems.**
  Sorting a problem into smaller parts can make the situation seem less overwhelming. Looking at each part of a problem helps you make a plan for each part.
- **Talk over important problems with others who tend to be levelheaded or who have been helpful in the past.**
  If you are feeling upset or discouraged, ask friends, neighbors, or family members to help. They can bring a calmer perspective to the situation as well as new ideas and help in dealing with the problems you are facing.

Anger

There are plenty of reasons to become angry when caring for an ill family member. Some people feel angry because their lives have been turned upside down by their caregiving responsibilities. The person they are caring for may, at times, be demanding and irritable. You may not feel appreciated. Sometimes people are angry because they are accustomed to fixing things, but cancer and its problems are not easily fixed. Friends, family members, or health professionals may not be as helpful or understanding as you would like.

These feelings are normal! It is all right to feel angry at times. It is how you deal with your anger that is important. Recognize your anger, accept it, and find some way to express it appropriately. If you do not deal with your anger, it can get in the way of almost everything you do.

Consider the following strategies for coping with anger:

- **Find safe ways to express your anger.**
  These outlets can include such things as beating on a pillow, yelling out loud in a car or in a closed room, or doing some vigorous exercise. Try writing down why you're so angry. Keep a diary and write down your feelings.
- **Talk with someone else about your anger in an appropriate way before it gets worse.**
  If you wait, your anger can lead you to say or do things you may later regret. Anger that is out of control can cloud your judgment. If possible, talk to someone outside the caregiving relationship about your anger before you talk to the person with cancer. Explaining to another person why you feel angry can help you understand the reasons for your feelings. Doing this first can also help you feel more prepared to talk to the person with cancer about the issue.
- **Get away from the situation for a while.**
  Go for a walk, a run, or go to a museum or movie for a while—whatever you need to do to remove yourself from the situation. Try to cool off before you go back and deal with what made you angry.

- ***Try to see the situation from the other person's point of view.***
  Recognize that other people are under stress, too, and some people are better than others at dealing with stressful situations.

Guilt

Many people caring for someone with cancer feel guilty at some time during the illness. They may feel guilty because they think they did something to cause the cancer or because they feel they should have recognized the cancer sooner. They may feel they should be doing a better job or may feel bad for taking time to look after their own needs. They may feel guilty because they are angry or upset with the person who has cancer. Caregivers also may feel guilty because they are healthy and the person they care about is sick. Perhaps they feel guilty about things that happened in the past that hurt their relationship with the person with cancer, and they wish they could change the past.

Although feeling guilty is understandable, it can interfere with your ability to do your best at caregiving. Guilt makes you focus only on your mistakes or shortcomings. Caregiving and relationships are two-way streets, and focusing only on one person's mistakes is not productive.

Consider the following strategies for coping with feelings of guilt:
- ***Talk to other people who have gone through similar experiences.***
  It is often easier to see a situation clearly when it is happening to someone else. Talking with someone else can give you perspective on your own problems.
- ***Don't expect to be perfect.***
  Expecting perfection of yourself can cause guilt to be a regular part of your life. It is helpful to remember that you are human. You will make mistakes from time to time. Accept them and move on.
- ***Don't dwell on mistakes.***
  Accept mistakes and get beyond them as best you can. The chapters on anxiety and depression in part II may further help you cope with feelings of guilt.

Fear

It is normal to be afraid when someone you care about has a serious illness. You do not know what is in store for either of you. You may be fearful that you will not be able to handle what happens.

Consider the following strategies for coping with fear:

- **Learn as much as possible about what is happening and what may happen in the future.**

  Learning more about the cancer, treatment, and prognosis of the person for whom you're caring can reduce the fear of the unknown. It can also help you to be realistic so that you can prepare for the future. Talk with health care professionals and with other people who have cared for someone with cancer to see whether you are exaggerating the risks and fears.

- **Talk to someone about your fears.**

  It often helps to explain your fears to an understanding person. This could be a friend or a mental health professional, such as a counselor. This process can help you think through the reasons for your feelings. Talking to a sympathetic person can also show you that other people understand and appreciate how you feel.

- **Read the chapter on anxiety (beginning on page 71).**

  The ideas and techniques in the chapter on anxiety can be used by you or the person with cancer to cope with feelings of fear.

Loss and sorrow

It can be very difficult to see physical or psychological changes in the person with cancer. Memories of how healthy and alert the person used to be may depress you. You may also feel unhappy because you have lost the normal, routine parts of your life that existed before the cancer. Perhaps you had plans for your future that are now in doubt.

Consider the following coping strategies for dealing with feelings of loss and sorrow:

- **Talk about your feelings of loss with other people who have had similar experiences.**

  People who have cared for a person with cancer will usually understand how you feel. Support groups are one way to find people who have had similar experiences and who can understand and appreciate your feelings. Some support groups can be found on the Internet. For example, go to the American Cancer Society Web site at **cancer.org**, and search for Cancer Survivors Network. This network has a special spot for family caregivers to chat with each other and support each other. You can also call **800-227-2345** to find a family caregiver support group that meets near you.

- **Read the chapter on depression (beginning on page 79).**

  Feelings of loss are often a part of feeling down or depressed. The ideas and techniques in the chapter on depression can help you to manage or prevent this condition.

⫸ Get help from others.

Don't try to do everything yourself. Caregiving can wear you out, increase your stress levels, and interfere with your ability to give good care at home. Ask for help. Consult the chapter "Getting Help from Community Agencies and Volunteer Groups" on pages 43–49 to learn about services such as support groups and home health care agencies that are available in your community. The resource guide at the end of this book will also help you locate assistance. Make arrangements for fill-in help from family members and friends. For example, you might ask for help driving the person to routine medical visits. Consider the following suggestions for making use of the people around you:

- *Try not to withdraw from family and friends, especially as caregiving gets more difficult.*

  Sometimes family caregivers don't feel like talking about their problems, or they're so busy that they don't find time to be with others. Caregivers, however, need to have social lives. Caregivers who have support from other people are less depressed and less overwhelmed by the responsibilities of caregiving. If you isolate yourself from others, you lose the stimulation, suggestions, and support that other people can provide.

- *Reach out to others and involve them in your life and in your caregiving.*

  This point is also important for the person with cancer. To achieve this goal, you need to make visits rewarding for visitors so they want to come again. Consider the following ways to involve others in caregiving:

  - *Make a list of people who can give companionship and support to you and the person with cancer.* Don't worry about how far away these people live, how busy they are, how long it has been since you talked to them, or even how well you know them. Make as long a list as possible so you have many choices.

  - *Go down your list, and for each person, think what you could do to make a visit (or a phone call) pleasant and enjoyable.* Use these ideas when you invite them and when they visit or call. This way they will want to come again, and you will feel good about asking them to return. For example, serve a nice snack or beverage. Show the visitor family pictures or cards. Suggest you all go on a short walk together.

  - *Have a list of ways that visitors can help in case they offer or if you feel comfortable asking.* Make your list specific so that people understand exactly what is needed. For example, your list might include tasks like taking out the trash, sweeping the porch, driving the person to treatment one day a week, or bringing in the mail. They will be able to budget their own time and be prepared to give the help you need.

Possible Challenges

Consider the following situations that have been difficult for other caregivers:

"He doesn't want to talk about feelings."

He is the best judge of that. Your job is to make sure the opportunities are there to share feelings when he decides the time is right.

"What if she talks about things that I don't want to hear?"

Even if what you hear hurts or upsets you, it may be helpful for her to express it. You don't have to solve anything. You're being helpful by just listening.

"He won't follow my advice."

Try to understand how important it is for him to retain some control. You may know what's best for him, but realize that your main job is support. Your job is not to make decisions for him. If you have a dominant personality or have been the one to make decisions in your family, you may have to give some of that control back to the person for whom you are caring.

"I'm swamped with problems, so I don't have time to take care of my needs."

This is the most common reason family caregivers become exhausted. They become preoccupied with problems and don't pay attention to themselves. You will be a better caregiver in the long run if you take the time, especially when stress is high, to get enough sleep, eat right, exercise, and do activities that you enjoy and that relax you.

"If I don't do it, it won't get done."

Sort out things that really need to be done versus what you would like to see done. It's okay to let some things, like housework, slide a bit when you take on new responsibilities. You can also ask family and friends for help instead of trying to do everything yourself.

"I hate to ask other people to help me."

There are a few ways around this problem. You can get together socially with people who could help and let them volunteer to help you, or you could have someone else ask them to help you. Try to remember that many people want to assist and simply don't know what to do. There is no shame in asking for help—others around you will then feel valuable and helpful.

"My father doesn't want other people to help us."

Suggest trying to get help for just a short time, such as for a week or even just a day. Then you can talk about how it worked. It also may be important to explain that you are the one who needs extra help, not him.

Carrying Out and Adjusting Your Plan

Think of other challenges that could interfere with carrying out your plan. What additional roadblocks could get in the way of your being an effective caregiver? Will the person for whom you are caring cooperate? How will you explain your needs to other people? Do you have the time and energy to carry out family caregiving responsibilities? Develop plans for getting around these challenges by using the COPE ideas discussed in the introduction.

Start using the ideas in this chapter now. Don't wait until you feel overwhelmed. It is easier to develop good caregiving habits and attitudes early before problems get out of hand. Set reasonable goals for yourself. It takes time and experience to improve your caregiving skills. Every week or so, take time to think about how you are doing as a caregiver. Reread this chapter periodically to get fresh ideas.

CHAPTER TWO

Helping Children Understand

A diagnosis of cancer creates changes and stress for all members of the family. It can be especially difficult for children. At the same time, it also can unite a family and be a stimulus for family members to help and support each other, especially by working together to solve problems. With support and help from adults, children can learn and grow emotionally through this difficult experience.

When to Get Professional Help

Some children may have difficulty adjusting to the situation and may need professional help to cope. Some behavior changes are normal when children hear disturbing news or when home routines are changed by cancer. If the behaviors are disruptive for the child and others and last more than a week or two, however, it is time to seek professional help. Look for the following signs that children are having trouble adjusting to changes caused by the cancer diagnosis:

- new negative or disruptive behaviors
- more frequent negative behaviors
- sleep disturbances lasting for more than a few days
- lack of normal appetite
- persistent physical complaints such as chest pains or stomach pains that lack a clear medical diagnosis
- new or sudden bed-wetting
- isolation or withdrawal that lasts and deepens
- increasing problems at school or skipping school
- loss of interest in what were previously normal activities, hobbies, or sports
- extreme perfectionism and fear of making mistakes
- displays of ritualistic behavior, such as frequent hand washing

- constant checking for reassurance, despite the presence of a supportive family
- making suicidal statements
- extreme compliance without self-expression

This last trait is less common and may be observed in children who normally behave well. They can suddenly become almost perfect—that is, they will be obedient, compliant, quiet, not express any feelings, and perhaps become more isolated and alone. This behavior may also include becoming more needy and clingy. These children, for example, may not want to leave their parents' sides.

Many families have not experienced this level of stress before now. Sometimes parents are so overwhelmed by the cancer diagnosis, the decisions to be made, and the challenges of treatment that they overlook a child's feelings. It may be helpful to talk to a doctor, a counselor, or a member of the clergy to help work out problems. Getting professional help is not a sign of weakness and is no reason to be embarrassed.

If you find you cannot discuss the issue openly or at all, consider seeking help from an outside source. This source might be a school guidance counselor, the child's teacher, hospital or clinic staff, or a cancer support group. One step many families take, even if they don't have difficulty talking about the disease, is to get counseling early in the cancer experience. You may find counseling helpful in heading off children's fears and anxieties. Again, people who might help include professional counselors, doctors or other medical staff members, hospital or clinic social workers, or members of the clergy.

Getting Help: Finding a Counselor

The logical place to start looking for help is at the center where the person with cancer receives treatment. Clinics and hospitals frequently offer support for people with cancer and their families. If help is not available at your treatment center and the staff there cannot offer guidance, ask your child's pediatrician or look at the resource guide at the back of this book.

Try to find someone with knowledge about children's reactions at varying ages and developmental levels—it could be a pediatrician, a child psychologist or psychiatrist, a social worker specializing in child and family issues, or a school guidance counselor.

What You Can Do

Coping with cancer can be an opportunity for strengthening family bonds. Families can often draw closer as they work together to overcome the stress and uncertainties of the illness. Try to keep these guidelines in mind for helping children understand and cope with what is happening:

- **Talk to the children about cancer,** telling them clearly what is going on and how it will affect the person with cancer and the rest of the family.
- **Listen to what the children say** about the illness and about what is going on in their lives, and encourage them to share their feelings.
- **Help children express their feelings.**
- **Involve the children** in the experience as much as is appropriate.
- **Continue to use rules of discipline and reward good behavior.**
- **Anticipate problems** children may have and try to deal with them before they become severe.

Talk to the Children About Cancer

There are many important reasons a child should be told that an adult in the household has cancer. First, children have an excellent ability to adapt to the truth. Even upsetting truths can be helpful in relieving their worry and anxiety about what is happening. In addition, children can learn they are important and needed by their family during times of stress. Children can help the person with cancer and give support during this difficult time. This situation may even help children learn to cope with stress and changes in their lives.

A child's security is built around routines and stability, and when those routines are threatened, the child may feel vulnerable. When an adult member of the household receives a cancer diagnosis, there are often changes in the routines, relationships, and experiences in the child's world. The appearance or energy levels of the person with cancer may change. Household schedules may change, and new people may be in the home. The distribution of household duties may change as well. All of these changes may affect the amount and kind of attention a child receives. Children need to understand why these changes happen and, as much as possible, they need stable routines.

For children, it is important that all adults be honest in order to maintain or foster trust. Children are observant and sensitive to changes in their loved ones. They can figure out that something is wrong without being told. They will notice facial expressions and tone of voice. They will overhear snatches of conversations. Without clear and honest communication, children will often create their own explanations for the changes, and their imaginations may paint a picture that is worse than reality.

Some of the following problems can occur when children are not informed:

- ***Children may create their own interpretation based on what they hear.***
  They may worry about getting cancer themselves, fear that no one will take care of them, or feel guilty, believing they did something to cause the illness.

- *Not talking about cancer may suggest that it is too terrible to discuss.*
  Not talking about cancer may actually increase the child's fear of the disease, rather than giving him or her comfort.
- *Children may find out the truth from someone else.*
  Hearing the truth from another source will only cause feelings of betrayal because those closest to them did not tell them first.
- *Fear may make things worse.*
  Fear of the unknown or that grown-ups are hiding something can make other problems—sleep or appetite problems, difficulties in school, withdrawal from family or friends, irritability, or fighting—even more difficult to resolve.

▐▶ **Be honest and clear when you break the news.**

Children, especially younger children, don't need to know everything about every test. However, if an adult family member receives a cancer diagnosis, tell the children soon—certainly before treatment begins.

Try to find a quiet place where you can talk without interruptions. Honesty and clarity are very important when telling a child about an adult's cancer. Keep in mind the brief attention span of younger children. Remember that especially for young children, feeling secure is important. Say something reassuring, such as, "We'll always love you, and we'll always be sure that you are cared for." At the very least, tell a young child the following details:

- **The diagnosis.** For example, you can say, *"Mom is sick with a disease called 'breast cancer.'"*
- **What treatments are expected, how they will affect the person, and how they might affect the young child.** For example, the person with cancer might say, *"I'm going to have surgery, which means removing the part of me that's not healthy. I won't be able to pick you up or hug you for a while, but you'll still be able to sit close to me."* The parent might tell the child, *"Grandpa has to take strong medicine that will make his hair fall out. He'll look different for a while, but he'll still be Grandpa."* Or the explanation might go, *"Dad is going to have less energy for a while. He'll need to rest more. We'll need to pick quiet times to do things together."*
- **The prognosis and chances of a cure.** You may choose to share this information only in response to direct questions from your child. If the prognosis is clearly very good, by all means, reassure the child: *"The doctors expect the treatment to get rid of the disease, so I will live a long time."* If the prognosis is less clear, focus on reassuring the child that someone will always be there. It is okay to be honest even if the prognosis may be unclear. For example, *"Dad is taking very strong medicine to get rid of the disease, and we hope it will make him better."*

Be aware that children have special needs at certain ages. If there are children of very different ages, you may want to talk with each of them separately or by age group. Preschoolers, for example, may feel overwhelmed or confused by too much information, while older children may want to learn as much as they can about cancer. The summary on pages 27–29 outlines children's expectations and needs for ages two to five, ages six to twelve, and for adolescents, along with information about what you can do to help children in each of these age groups cope with the illness of a parent or loved one.

No matter the child's age, it's important for the adult to be a careful listener and ask the child what he or she wants to know. Answer questions clearly and honestly. Especially with younger children, it is useful to give only the information the child asks for, using a vocabulary matched to the child's age level.

Listen to What the Children Say

Almost everything revolves around communication. Keep the lines of communication open between adults and children. Even if what children say is upsetting, continue to encourage them to share openly. Talk to them about changes that are happening as a result of the illness. Children often find it difficult to share their feelings. If your child seems to have trouble, your goal should be to help the child express him- or herself. You may need to say, "Other kids have feelings like this, and it's okay to feel afraid or angry—it's important to share feelings." Sometimes it helps just to recognize that problems are going on in the family and talk about it.

Talking about a child's fear that a beloved adult may die is an especially sensitive topic. Keep in mind that if a child asks about the person dying, he or she may really be asking something else. The child may be concerned about what will happen to the family or what will happen to him or her if a parent dies. Children often communicate things indirectly, and it may be up to you to open the lines of communication and feelings.

Help Children Express Their Feelings

There are a variety of ways to help children express their feelings:

▦➡ **Encourage young children to express their feelings through art.**
Young children can be encouraged to draw a picture of their feelings. Emotions can be given names and assigned colors; for example, red can represent anger, yellow can be happiness, blue can be sadness, and black can be fear. Ask the child to color a circle that shows how much he or she is feeling angry, happy, sad, scared, and so on.

▦▶ Consider a "feelings bag" to help young, school-age children talk about their feelings.

Elementary school–age children are beginning to understand the differences between feelings they show and those they keep inside. A paper grocery bag can become a "feelings bag." On the outside, the child can draw or glue pictures that represent feelings that others see. On the inside of the bag, the child can place pictures that he or she is less comfortable sharing with others.

▦▶ Consider play-acting and role-playing to help children express thoughts and fears.

Dramatic role-playing can help children express feelings to others. Try switching roles. Ask the child to pretend to be the person with cancer while you take turns as the doctor, the child, or other people who are involved. If older children are worried about how to talk to peers, volunteer to play the friend while the child practices telling the friend about the illness.

▦▶ Use storytelling with young elementary school–age children as a way to talk about fears and clear up misunderstandings.

Rather than reading a bedtime story, suggest that you make up a story together. You can begin by creating an imaginary family similar to your own. Once the story is under way, it is the child's turn to continue the story. You and the child can weave the story together, and you can provide support and solutions for problems the child identifies through the story.

▦▶ Encourage preteens and teenagers to talk openly.

He or she may want to learn as much as possible about the disease. Adolescents may be helped by attending a support group of their peers or visiting an online support group to hear how others are coping with the same issues. Some treatment centers conduct groups specifically for teenagers. Keeping a diary or writing a story about the family may also help. Help direct teens to reputable Web sites—whereas there is a great deal of information on the Internet, not all of that information is reliable. See the resource guide at the back of this book for a list of reliable resources, including some directed at teenagers.

▦▶ Make a conscious effort to be available to the children during this illness.

Dedicate a specific amount of time you will spend with the child on a regular basis. It is natural for adults to focus on the illness and the problems of the person with cancer. Establishing a time (daily or weekly) to spend with the child will go a long way toward keeping communication open. This time should be free of interruptions or TV, a time when you can just ask, "How are you doing?" or "How has your day been?" It is important to talk both about the child's feelings related to the cancer and about the other things going on in his or her life.

⦚➡ **Plan how the person with cancer will communicate with the children when not at home.**

The person with cancer may have to travel for treatment or may have to stay in the hospital sometimes. You can sustain communication by talking on the phone, sending notes, e-mailing, and making recorded messages.

⦚➡ **Avoid trying to protect children by not sharing such feelings as anger, fear, or worry.**

Failing to share negative feelings may have a negative impact. It may communicate to children that such feelings are unacceptable or abnormal. They may then feel guilty when they have these feelings. A better approach is to share your feelings and how you are coping with those feelings. You may tell the child, for example, "I feel very angry that this has happened to us. Sometimes at night I pound my pillow to let the anger out." Or you might say, "Mom was feeling very scared about her treatments, but the doctors and nurses have helped us see the treatments as the strong medicine she needs to get rid of the disease."

⦚➡ **Avoid discussing aspects of treatment that are especially scary to children.**

If, for example, needles frighten a child, think about what you'll say when you describe the treatment, and minimize what you say about injections. It is a natural tendency to describe in great detail experiences that are new or difficult. It is better to save those descriptions for adults who are better able to understand and give you support.

⦚➡ **Use humor to defuse tensions.**

Allowing children to laugh and joke about the situation can lighten the emotional load. For example, some people who have a prosthesis give it a name. You are the best judge for what will work for your family, but don't be afraid to use humor.

Involve the Children

Try to involve the children as much as is appropriate. Encourage children to help, and let them discuss changes to their routines.

⦚➡ **Suggest things children can do around the house.**

These tasks will differ among age groups, but everybody can do something to help. Even a two-year-old can give Mommy a hug, and teenagers can help with adult chores. Whatever the task, each child should feel that he or she is contributing and helping the family get through this crisis. These contributions can help children have a sense of control and participation in their surroundings.

▐▶ **Sit down as a family and discuss some of the changes that may occur.**
Change can be very stressful for children. Changes are less scary, however, if you and your family know to expect them. Part of the child's role in the family is to help cope with changes, which will be easier if the changes are expected.

▐▶ **Look for opportunities to create rituals and continue old ones.**
Rituals can provide stability in children's lives during difficult periods. These rituals should be pleasant activities the child can count on and should not require much effort on the part of the adults. It might be a weekly movie night with popcorn or takeout or a weekly sleepover at a grandparent's or neighbor's house. During periods of separation, it could be a phone call from the person with cancer every morning.

▐▶ **Include older children in the treatment experience.**
Bring older, school-age children along to an appointment. Doctors and nurses can answer any questions the child may have. This visit will also allow the child to see the hospital or clinic as a friendly and supportive environment, rather than a bad place where people do mean things. If the person with cancer is going to be hospitalized, children should be prepared for what they will see, hear, and smell during hospital visits.

ADOLESCENT DAUGHTERS OF MOTHERS WITH BREAST CANCER

Adolescence can be a time when communication between mothers and daughters is strained. The stress of a mother receiving a diagnosis of breast cancer can add to that strain. Mothers may need more assistance from their daughters. Daughters may be very uncomfortable talking about issues related to breasts if they are undergoing breast development.

Both mother and daughter may have concerns about the daughter's risk of breast cancer because of the mother's cancer diagnosis. Doctors are gaining a much better understanding of breast cancer risk within families. Chances are the daughter's risk is only slightly increased from that of other women and standard screening is still appropriate. Make sure the daughter is instructed in breast self-examination as she nears the end of adolescence. If the doctor thinks the family history suggests a genetic breast cancer, the family may want to look for a clinic that specializes in breast cancer risk assessment. If the doctor is not aware of this resource, contact your American Cancer Society at **800-227-2345** or call the National Cancer Institute's Cancer Information Service at **800-422-6237**.

Continue To Use Rules of Discipline and Reward Good Behavior

Continuing to enforce family rules and reward good behavior can help children feel more secure.

➠ **Continue to set limits on negative behaviors.**

Discipline can be difficult to enforce when children act up or behave badly as a way of coping with the stresses of a family illness. A breakdown in rules, however, can convince children that things are really wrong and add to their feelings of insecurity. Tell children that you love them but will not accept destructive or bad behavior.

➠ **Whenever possible, use rewards rather than punishments to guide and manage a child's behavior.**

Displace bad behavior by rewarding good behavior that takes its place. Consistency in both rewards and punishments can help children feel secure and know their world is under control. Examples of good behaviors are sharing feelings in positive ways, helping other family members, cooperating with others, being responsible for schoolwork and household chores, and showing consideration and care for adults.

Anticipate Problems

Changes in a child's behavior may indicate a problem. Some children may not want to separate from an adult and may be clingy out of a sense of fear. If this happens, it may be important to talk about feelings of fear. Some children avoid their feelings by being silly and acting goofy. Such behavior may be a cue that the child is having difficulty facing his or her feelings. Some children stay away from the person with cancer because they are afraid their loved one will die. If these behaviors occur, talk to the child about the importance of getting through this difficult and scary time together.

➠ **Pay attention to age group issues.**

Children of different ages and developmental levels have different expectations and needs. These are some of the thoughts and concerns that are common in children, separated here into three broad age groupings—toddlers and young children, elementary school–age children, and adolescents.

Possible issues for toddlers and young children (ages 2 to 5)
- fear of being separated from a parent or someone they love
- fear of "catching" the disease
- thinking they caused the illness by misbehaving
- becoming angry because they receive less attention

- confusion about the disease, its cause, treatments, and what it does to the person with cancer

Ways to help

Be honest. Don't exceed the child's attention span, and repeat and reinforce messages of security and love for the child. Try to limit the number of caretakers for the child. Reassure the child that cancer is not contagious and that he or she did not cause the person to become sick.

Possible issues for elementary and early middle school–age children (ages 6 to 12)
- fear of changes in family, lifestyles, activities, and security
- fear of embarrassment over being different from friends and possible guilt over being embarrassed
- need for details about the person's condition and treatment
- fear of "catching" the disease
- anger over limitations imposed on them by the illness
- confusion about how to explain the illness to friends
- questioning of the role of religion

Ways to help

Be clear that cancer is not contagious and that the children did not cause the person's cancer. Let children know in advance about babysitters or caretakers who may come in to watch them. Keep the child's school informed about the family's situation. It may help to have the child come along to treatment or to talk with the doctors and nurses who are taking care of the person with cancer.

Possible issues for adolescents
- resentment and/or fear over changes in family, lifestyles, and activities
- sensitivity to deception—any deception will cause distrust at this age, and you should tell the truth at all costs
- feeling guilty about wanting to exert independence at a time when they are needed at home
- embarrassment over being different from peers or over the physical appearance of the person with cancer
- confusion over what may happen
- conflicted feelings because the illness reinforces their lack of control at a time when they want and expect more control over their lives
- questioning of the role or validity of religion

For adolescents, rapid and confusing change is already a part of their lives as they make the transition from dependent children to independent adults. The additional confusion and change that comes from a serious illness in the family only adds to their stress.

Ways to help

Adolescents sometimes feel more comfortable talking to someone outside of their families about their feelings. This could be a friend, teacher, counselor, or other trusted adult. Keep the school informed of the family's situation. Show your willingness to talk about religion, even if his or her feelings or thoughts are challenging. Encourage adolescents to maintain hobbies, sports, or other activities. Be careful not to load down adolescents with too much responsibility. They are not yet adults. Give them some breathing room.

Possible Challenges

Consider the following situations that have been difficult for other caregivers:

"My mother-in-law has given up on my wife and talks about her as if death is just a matter of time. I can see that my son is taking this in and getting more and more worried."
A good response to your mother-in-law would be, "Please don't think that everyone who has cancer is going to die," and explain to her what you've told your son. You might write a brief letter that explains tactfully but frankly your approach to helping your son understand the situation. Outline exactly what you want your son to know and ask that the grandmother respect this approach and not contradict your message. You might also arrange for your child to talk to the doctor. Tell the child, for example, that his grandmother does not have all the information.

"Megan overheard us discussing how strapped we are for finances with all of the medical bills we're getting. She's started to think we may be losing our house."
When children overhear talk about money worries, they tend to think the worst—that they are not going to have any food or a home. This concern also applies to discussions about who will take care of your child. You may be talking about arranging for someone to be with your child tomorrow afternoon when you go for treatment, but the child may misunderstand and think you are planning a caretaker for after the parent's death. Discussions about the logistics of arranging childcare can also lead a young child to feel abandoned, unwanted, and unloved.

Reassure your children that you love them and they do not need to worry about whether they will be cared for. Be very conscious of what you say in front of your children or in places where they can overhear. If your house is small or a child's bedroom is right over the dining room where you sit and talk, try to find another place to talk.

"What if I break down and cry when we tell our children about their Dad's cancer? What if I don't handle all of this perfectly?"

It is okay and healthy for children to see that their parents have feelings. While it can be upsetting to young children to see their parents upset, it can also be good for them to see that feelings are normal and healthy. Even if you or your husband does lose control and break down, you're still the best people to talk with your children.

"What about the other kids at school? How will they react to my child when they learn her mother has cancer?"

Children's friends and schoolmates can be supportive or destructive. They may spread rumors, and they may tell your child things like, "Well, Joey's mother died, so your mother will, too." Your job is to talk honestly with your child about the specifics of your situation, based on the child's age and maturity level. Tell your child that some children might say things that are different from what you've said, but that they are not the authority. Emphasize that you will always tell them the truth and that their friends do not have all of the facts.

In addition, you can try involving teachers, guidance counselors, or coaches. You can ask them to encourage the child's peers to be supportive. Sometimes children say cruel or thoughtless things merely because they lack experience—nobody has ever told them how to be a supportive friend to a child whose mother has cancer.

If your child is an adolescent, you might ask whether it is okay if you answer his or her peers directly if they ask questions.

"Between my job, taking my wife to clinic appointments, and running to the pharmacy to get her medicine, it seems that my son and I are like ships passing in the night. As soon as I get back from the doctor's office, Sean is leaving for baseball practice. When he gets home, I'm exhausted and ready for bed."

The demands of daily living can drain the energy of a family caregiver, as well as the person with cancer. Make sure that once a day or once a week, you do something together as a family and talk together as a family. It is important to establish some time together that won't be interrupted.

Carrying Out and Adjusting Your Plan

Think of other challenges that could interfere with your plan to help your child understand and adjust to the changes taking place at home. What additional roadblocks could get in the way of following the recommendations in this chapter? Will the person with cancer cooperate? Will other people support your approach and not contradict your message? How will you explain your family's situation to schools or other childcare providers? Do you have the time and energy to carry out your plan? Develop plans for getting around these challenges using the COPE ideas discussed in the introduction.

A weekly check-in with each child is a good idea, just to ask some questions: How are you doing? Are you having any problems in school? For school issues, periodically talk with your child's teachers and others who interact with your child to keep them aware of the situation, ask how your child is doing, and to ask them to continue watching for major changes in behavior or mood.

One way you can evaluate how things are going is to look at whether the child is able to continue with normal daily routines. For example, the daily routine of a four-year-old might be saying good-bye to Mom, going to preschool, and playing. If your child is in sixth grade, he or she needs to be able to go to school, do assignments, and interact with friends. Children need some normality—they need to be able to pursue the "work" of their lives and to talk to you about their experiences.

Reactions to an illness can happen at any time. Some children display behavioral problems early in the illness, whereas others show problems later. Sometimes children begin to misbehave after their parents are past the worst phases of cancer diagnosis and treatment and are starting to feel better. With parental help, most children cope well throughout most of the illness, and most grow to be stronger people because of it.

CHAPTER THREE

Coordinating Care from One Treatment Setting to Another

People with cancer are usually in the hospital more than once during different episodes of their illnesses. They also may spend time in a rehabilitation center or nursing home. Caregivers may need to be ready to help a patient transition from a hospital or other health care facility to the home, and he or she may also have to facilitate the opposite: transitioning the routines and methods you've developed at home into a new health care facility. Other times, the person may need to move from one medical environment to another, such as from a hospital to a rehabilitation facility. As you work out routines and schedules and learn to manage different symptoms and problems, you will want to see many of these same routines followed as closely as possible wherever the person is.

When to Get Professional Help

If the problems in coordinating care are making the person with cancer very uncomfortable and you have tried the ideas in this chapter without success, ask to speak to a nurse supervisor or physician. Explain the problems you are having and why you are concerned. If you still have problems, ask to talk to the patient advocate at the hospital. Patient advocates are on the staff of most hospitals, and their job is to help when you feel the hospital is not doing its job.

What You Can Do

This chapter will discuss what you can do to help ease transitions in three different types of situations:

- **transitioning the patient from a hospital environment to the home,**
- **transitioning from home to a hospital environment, and**
- **coordinating the transition from one medical environment to another.**

Transitioning from Hospital to Home

Taking someone home from the hospital can be challenging, especially if he or she has new medicines, has had new procedures, is weak as a result of surgery or treatment, or needs help with everyday tasks, such as bathing. Ideally, the hospital social worker or case manager should meet with you to discuss what kinds of help you may need at home. There may be situations, however, in which the person is released and you have not yet met with a social worker. Skilled nursing care can be arranged by the doctor or nurse through a home health care agency, but nurses from a home health care agency may not be able to come to the home on the day the patient is released. In these situations, you and the person with cancer may be faced with solving some home care problems on your own. There are a number of things you can do to help prepare for the transition to home:

▸ **Bring home the phone numbers of local home health care agencies who can send a registered nurse to the house, ideally the day after hospital discharge.**
If the staff tells you to call home health care agencies for help when you get home, ask the staff for the phone numbers and get them before you leave the hospital. Try to coordinate with the home health care agency as soon as possible, so that there is no delay in the nurse's visit to the house.

▸ **Arrange to have extra help when you arrive home to get the person up or down any steps.**
When the person comes home from the hospital, he or she may need help getting out of the car and walking up or down any steps. Having a friend or family member to help with this task prevents you from struggling and risking a fall.

▸ **Make sure you understand the person's medication regimen.**
Pain control can be a key factor in successful home care. Talk to the person's health care team to be sure you understand all of the person's medication needs.

▸ **Ask whether the hospital pharmacy can fill prescriptions before you leave.**
Leaving the hospital with any necessary prescription medicines will save you time and ensure the pills are ready when the person with cancer needs them.

▸ **Ask whether a local pharmacy can deliver medicines to the home in a pill box.**
Some pharmacies will deliver medicines to the home, and many will even organize medicines in a pill box, where the pills are placed in the time slot when they need to be taken for each day of the week. Even if delivery is not available, the pharmacy may still be able to provide the person's

medicine in a pill box. Ask for a "medi-set," medication box, or pill box when you get medicines. Having a pill box means that you and the person with cancer have one less thing to do: figure out what pills need to be taken when.

IIII➡ **Get detailed instructions from the person's doctor regarding warning symptoms or signs that could indicate a worsening condition.**
Make sure you know what to do and/or whom to contact should the person get worse.

IIII➡ **Arrange for a walker or wheelchair, if needed.**
If the person is weak, he or she can lean on a walker or sit in a wheelchair to get from one place to another. Hospital staff can help you arrange for these types of equipment ahead of time if you ask. Wheelchairs and walkers are available at medical supply stores and some pharmacies, and the stores may be able to deliver them. Health insurance may cover the cost of the equipment if you get a doctor's order.

IIII➡ **Arrange for a hospital bed, if needed.**
If the person with cancer needs a hospital bed, he or she will also qualify for visits from home health care nurses. These nurses can arrange for a bed. These are usually rented and covered by your health insurance with a doctor's order. They also can be purchased. The benefit of a hospital bed is that the person can sit up for meals or beverages in bed without having to get out of bed. It can also be helpful because the person can sit up before trying to get out of bed. In addition, if the person has problems with breathing, raising the bed can help ease breathing problems. These beds are usually electric, which saves your bending to use a crank to raise the head or foot of the bed. An electric bed also makes it easier for the person with cancer to adjust his or her position independently.

IIII➡ **Arrange for oxygen at home, if needed.**
Many people live comfortably at home with oxygen. Tanks are delivered by a respiratory therapy company. Adults at home are taught how to use the equipment, how to recognize when more oxygen tanks are needed, how to replace the tanks, and how to solve problems with the oxygen delivery.

IIII➡ **Plan for a ride home.**
It may sound simple, but sometimes hospital discharges happen suddenly. You may not have time to arrange for someone to drive the person with cancer home, and you may not be able to drive the person home by yourself. Think about this the day after the person with cancer goes to the hospital so you have some ideas about whom to call ahead of time if you are not driving.

The person with cancer may have arrived at the hospital in an ambulance but going home in one is expensive and not always the best option.

➡ **Get instructions for caring for the person's ostomy or catheter, if applicable.**
If the person has an ostomy or catheter, you may be able to help him or her care for it or you may need the help of a home health care agency or visiting nurse. Be sure you understand what is required.

➡ **Decide whether a bedside portable commode is needed.**
When a person is weak, getting from a bed or chair to the bathroom can be a long walk. Having a commode at the bedside makes it easier for the person to get to the toilet. Bedside portable commodes are available through medical equipment stores and covered by health insurance if you have a doctor's order. They can sometimes be purchased at pharmacies.

➡ **Take a urinal home for men to use in bed or from a chair.**
A male urinal is plastic and is easily washed out. Using a male urinal can limit the number of times the man has to get up and walk to the bathroom.

Transitioning from Home to Hospital

Telling the health care staff what works at home helps them offer the best possible care in their setting. If you do not inform the health care staff, particularly the admitting physician, about the person's needs and routines, then the person with cancer may, as a consequence, have unmanaged symptoms. For example, if you have established a schedule of pain pills that keeps the pain away and also keeps him or her fully alert, you will want the person to stay on this dosing schedule when hospitalized. Changes to the dosing schedule could happen if the person is admitted to a different hospital from the one where the doctor who prescribed the pain medicine works. Changes could also occur if a different doctor prescribes additional doses of pain medicine. The person with cancer might have been treated by medical oncologists for months but be seen later by a radiation oncologist and given a higher dose of pain medicine. If the person returns to the medical oncologist, the new pain prescriptions need to be explained. The doctor or nurse admitting the person to the hospital needs to know exactly what medicines are given at home, when they are given, and how effective they are.

Maintaining medication schedules is not the only concern. Equipment that works well at home (such as a certain walker or toilet seat) should be used in the hospital. Personal care preferences and routines should be stated and followed in the new care setting, if possible. Your goal as caregiver is to continue effective routines as the person with cancer moves from one treatment setting to another.

First, consider what kinds of personal help is needed with such tasks as taking medicines or eating; help with medical procedures, such as caring for an ostomy or catheter; mobility issues such as getting out of bed or walking; sleeping; or personal hygiene, including toileting and bathing. Does the person have any other special needs?

Take some time to prepare answers to the following questions.

- Is any special equipment needed, such as a commode or special mattress?
- Is the person on a special diet? Are there food likes or dislikes?
- What kinds of things make the day more enjoyable for him or her, such as listening to music, watching television, talking on the phone, reading the newspaper, or getting the mail?
- What does he or she worry about, and how can the staff be most comforting and reassuring?
- What other facts would you want to tell those who will be involved in caregiving? For example, is he or she a smoker? Is there a need for help withdrawing from the nicotine in cigarettes, such as a nicotine patch, antidepressants, or other medicine?

For a person transitioning from home to hospital, his or her needs can be grouped into two categories: continuing medical care and continuing familiar routines.

⟫ Continue medical schedules and routines.

Plan how you can continue the same schedules and routines to prevent distressing symptoms or discomfort.

- *Give a medicine list to the admitting doctor or nurse, including the names of medicines and times of day those medicines are given.*

  Putting the medicine schedule in writing ensures that medicines can be given close to the same times as usual. It is especially important to do this step for medicines that were originally ordered to be given as needed, or "prn." If you give the medication schedule to the admitting doctor or nurse, he or she can ensure that the routine changes as little as possible. See table 3.1 for an example.

- *List any food or liquid that is given with medications in the medication schedule.*

  The staff can then write in their plans "give with milk" or "serve with a small amount of applesauce."

- *Write down the form in which medications are given.*

  For example, the pill might be crushed or mixed with applesauce or simethicone (Maalox) or other gas relief medicine. Perhaps the medicine is given as a rectal suppository. Write down instructions so there will be no confusion.

- ***Ask the admitting doctor and nurse to follow the home elimination routine if the person has not had a bowel movement.***

  Unfortunately, it often takes a few days to notice constipation at a new setting. If the person has not had a bowel movement and you would typically give a laxative or enema at home, ask the admitting doctor to follow that same routine. If the same elimination routine is followed, less discomfort will result.

- ***Ask the doctors and nurses to write the bowel elimination routine, medication requirements, and any other key information in the nursing care plan.***

  Many times the family gives key information to the doctor or nurse who admits the person, but it is written down in a long admission note, which may not be read by doctors or nursing staff on other shifts. If key information is written on the medical orders and in the nursing care plan, it will be noticed and used in caring for the patient.

- ***Ask the nurses to order a bedside commode or raised toilet seat if either was used at home.***

  If the person has been using a bedside commode or raised toilet seat, it will likely to be needed in the new setting, too. Tell the admitting physician or nurse about this need so that the right equipment is available.

- ***Ask the doctor to order a soft or blender-processed diet if it is preferred.***

  Ordering a soft diet ensures that meals are edible if a sore mouth, mucositis, or mouth ulcers are a problem.

Table 3.1. Sample Medication Chart to Give to Admitting Nurse or Doctor				
MEDICINE	**HOW MUCH/ HOW OFTEN**	**WHEN**	**WHAT FORM**	**TAKE HOW/ WITH WHAT**
AMOXICILLIN	250 mg/ every 8 hours	8:00 a.m. 4:00 p.m. 12:00 a.m.	Tablet	Crush tablet in small amount of applesauce.
PHENERGAN	25 mg/ every 4–6 hours	As needed	Rectal suppository	Give before meals.
TAMOXIFEN	10 mg/ twice a day	10:00 a.m. 5:00 p.m.	Tablet	Give with large glass of water.

- **Ask the doctor to write the mouth care regimen in the admitting orders.**

  If warm salt rinses or baking soda rinses are routine at home, ask that they be included in the doctor's admitting orders and the nursing care plan so that staff will give these items to the person and help with rinsing. Otherwise, it will be up to you or the person for whom you are caring to bring in salt or baking soda and remember to rinse after meals and at bedtime.

⟱➤ **Continue familiar routines.**

There are many ways to continue familiar routines in a new environment:

- **Bring the mail and newspaper from home.**

  Familiar routines are not limited to medicines and personal care. Staying in touch with one's home can also bring a sense of comfort and control.

- **Bring a radio and music or relaxation recordings.**

  Distractions, no matter how short, are important for relief of the anxiety and tension that can go along with being in the hospital or nursing center. Music can be brought in and played for enjoyment and distraction. Radios are not usually available in these settings, so you may have to bring one in for the person to listen to favorite news or music programs. Headphones can be used if the person is in a semiprivate room.

- **Bring turbans, scarves, caps, or head coverings worn at home.**

  Appearance can be very important to someone who is sick.

- **Bring in aids for walking, such as canes or walkers.**

- **Bring in aids for comfort and sleep, such as small pillows or favorite blankets.**

- **Ask ahead for a special mattress if one is needed.**

  Many people like the feel and contour of foam eggshell mattresses. Other mattresses are filled with air or water and may be more comfortable if skin care is a problem. If a special mattress is used at home, ask that the same type be used in the new setting. If you ask ahead of time, it is more likely to be available when the person is admitted. Even if it isn't, asking beforehand may help in getting it sooner.

- **Make sure the person can get to the telephone easily and has important telephone numbers available.**

  It is important for the person to be able to communicate with friends and family if that is part of the normal routine and if he or she is able.

Transitioning From One Medical Setting to Another

Sometime the person with cancer is transferred from one hospital to another or to a rehabilitation facility or long-term care setting, such as a nursing home. In this situation, plan how you can continue the same routines and schedules to prevent distressing symptoms or discomfort.

➠ **Work with admitting staff at a new facility to ensure continuity in medications and care routines.**

Be sure the staff at the new facility know when medications should be given, as well as in what form and whether any specific foods or beverages are given with the medicines.

➠ **Work with admitting staff to be sure preferred equipment is used.**

If the person needs any special equipment, such as a portable toilet, walker, or special mattress, speak with the staff as soon as possible to request that equipment.

➠ **Work with admitting staff to ensure bowel elimination routine is followed.**

As discussed earlier, it can sometimes take a few days to notice constipation in a new setting. Try to adhere to the same elimination routine as in the previous setting.

➠ **Make sure you understand the plan of care.**

Speak with the health care team at the transferring facility and follow up with the staff at the new facility to ensure clear communications. Transitions between facilities can be complicated, and it is important to ensure that both you and the relevant medical staff are on the same page regarding the person's overall condition and care.

Possible Challenges

Consider the following situations that have been difficult for other caregivers:

"Won't the doctor coordinate care?"

Doctors may not know which routines have been effective at home or in other treatment settings. You have to tell them. Give the doctor a list of medicines, how they are taken (such as pills, suppositories, or injections), times they are taken, and a list of what helps the person swallow medicine (see table 3.1). Doctors also don't know the specific bowel elimination plan, mouth care routines, diets, or equipment that helps the person with cancer at home. If you ask the doctor to write this information as medical orders, the nurses will follow these orders.

"I don't want the staff to think I'm bossing them around."

Nurses and doctors will welcome your input. Information about the person's care is important for the person's comfort and health. Writing important information down will make it easier for the staff to include this information in the medical record.

40   American Cancer Society

"They don't have enough staff to do all the things I am asking for."

You have a right to expect good care. If your requests are important for the person's health and comfort, they should be taken into consideration. You may have to speak up if you don't feel your requests are being honored. You may also have to visit often to be sure these routines are being followed. Care should never be compromised because of insufficient staffing.

Carrying Out and Adjusting Your Plan

Think of other possible challenges that could interfere with coordinating care from one treatment setting to another. What additional roadblocks could get in the way of following the recommendations in this chapter? Will the medical staff cooperate? How will you explain what is needed to care providers in new settings? Do you have the time and energy to carry out the plan? Develop plans for getting around these challenges by using the COPE ideas discussed in the introduction.

If possible, write down your requests before the person goes to a new treatment setting and give the instructions to the staff before the transfer occurs. If the transfer happens too quickly for this to be possible, take your lists to the new medical staff as soon as you can.

If the person for whom you are caring is in a hospital or other facility, ask whether your requests are being accommodated. Ask the nurses to see a copy of their orders, and check to be sure your requests are included. If you are having difficulty getting the information to the right person or the staff is not following your wishes, ask another staff member to help you. Involve this person in solving the problem of coordinating care. Social workers are often good sources of help. They know the doctors and nurses and can give them your lists and ideas.

If you still are unhappy about how care is being handled, ask to speak with the head nurse or patient advocate. Patient advocates are on the staff of most hospitals, and their job is to help resolve issues with patients' care. Such steps are usually not needed, however, as health care staff will likely want to continue using any methods that worked at home.

CHAPTER FOUR

Getting Help from Community Agencies and Volunteer Groups

Many people with cancer and their families do not fully understand the support services that are available to them in their own communities and in the hospitals or clinics where they receive treatment. As a result, they struggle alone with problems when there are people and organizations able and willing to help. Finding out about these services and how to qualify for and use them can be a challenge.

This chapter discusses the types of services that people with cancer sometimes need: help with transportation and driving, home nursing visits, and help with meals and household chores. These services are available in most communities.

We recommend you learn about available services before problems arise. This will mean learning whom to ask about community services, what services are available in your community or hospital, and how to qualify for and use those helpful services. Even if you don't need the services yet, knowing they are available is like having money in the bank. It can be reassuring to know that there are resources available if you need them. It is also easier to learn about these services when you are not under pressure to deal with a serious problem. When and if you need support services, you will know what to do and where to go immediately.

When to Get Professional Help

If you are having difficulty arranging the help you need, ask to speak to a social worker or caseworker. Social workers and caseworkers are experienced in finding help through community agencies and volunteer groups. Most hospitals have social workers or caseworkers on their staff or can refer you to a social services organization for assistance. Ask a doctor or nurse at the hospital to arrange for you to talk to a social worker or caseworker.

What You Can Do

- **Find the services available.**
- **Arrange transportation and driving, as necessary.**
- **Arrange home nursing services, as necessary.**
- **Find help with meals and household chores, as necessary.**

Find the Services Available

There are a number of places you can go for help in finding and using services in the community. We suggest you try all of these options; one resource may list a service that others do not. See also the section on caregiver resources in the resource guide beginning on page 299.

➤ **Ask social workers or caseworkers at your hospital or clinic.**

Social workers and caseworkers have knowledge, skills, and experience in finding community services to help people with cancer and their families deal with illness-related problems. They deal regularly with community agencies and know what services are available and which agencies provide the best service. You are entitled to talk with hospital social workers if the person is being treated at the hospital, either on an inpatient or outpatient basis. You can usually call the social worker directly without being referred, but some hospitals prefer that the doctor refer your case to the social worker. Talk to your doctor or nurse to determine the best way to proceed. If a knowledgeable social worker is not available, ask an oncology nurse to help you instead.

➤ **Ask knowledgeable people in your community.**

Some community members will be great sources of information about which local agencies and organizations provide services. Clergy are usually well informed on these matters, as are local elected officials and officers of local community organizations, such as the United Way. If these people cannot help you directly, they usually know whom to ask.

➤ **Search out agencies that can help locate services.**

Most communities have agencies that specialize in helping people find services they need. They have different titles in different communities or parts of the country, but these groups include the United Way, the Area Agency on Aging, religious agencies (such as Catholic Charities or the local Council of Churches), and community mental health centers. Hospital social workers are a good source of information about agencies in your area and can explain what services they provide. To learn more about resources in your area, you can also contact your American Cancer Society at **800-227-2345** or visit the Web site at **cancer.org**.

➡ **Look in the telephone book or online for social or human services (or a section with a similar title, if looking in the phone book) for agencies in your area.**
Most local telephone books contain sections listing community agencies and the services they provide. This listing may be in a separate section and be printed on paper of a different color (often blue). Look at the table of contents in the beginning of your local telephone book for the human services or community services section. Also see pages 299–318 for a list of resources for caregivers.

Arrange Transportation and Driving, as Necessary

Getting transportation to and from treatments or medical appointments can be difficult. Look for help if any of the following conditions exist:

- You cannot drive the person to appointments.
- You cannot get the person from the house to the car, or the person cannot sit upright for the length of the trip.
- You fear falling asleep at the wheel, the trip is too long, you hesitate to drive, or you are anxious about making the trip.
- You cannot miss work or cannot afford to take time off for the trip.

Possible solutions to transportation problems require asking for help, but many sources are available.

➡ **Ask family or friends for help with driving.**
The more specific you are about what you need, the more likely it is that others will understand your request and be able to judge what services they could provide. Tell them the following specific information:

- the day(s) of the week you need drivers
- the length of the trip
- whether the person can be dropped off
- whether someone will meet the person with cancer at the door
- the costs for parking
- how long the average appointment lasts
- whether the person needs help getting in and out of the vehicle.
- whether a wheelchair is involved
- whether money is available to pay for gas

➡ **Ask a family member or friend to arrange transportation, either from an agency or from another friend or family member.**
If you don't want to ask for help, have someone else ask for you. Having another person act as

the scheduler is especially helpful when the person with cancer must go for treatment every day or every week. For example, church groups often arrange transportation for members and may be willing to arrange drivers for nonmembers.

➠ **Contact your American Cancer Society at 800-227-2345 and ask whether they have a volunteer transportation program.**
Many offices of the American Cancer Society run transportation programs. Volunteer drivers are trained to help the person with cancer, and the service is free. In addition, the schedule of drivers is arranged for you. If your local office does not have such a program, ask whether the next closest office has a transportation program. Sometimes volunteer drivers who live slightly farther away (for example, the next county) are willing to help with driving. If your local American Cancer Society office does not have a driver available, it may still be able to help you locate one.

➠ **Ask local service clubs, such as the Elks, Lions Club, Masons, or American Legion, whether they are able to schedule drivers, help with transportation expenses, or help locate transportation assistance.**
A number of other organizations have volunteers who drive people with serious illnesses to medical appointments. This service varies from community to community. Some service groups raise money to help with medical or transportation expenses. If a relative or friend belongs to such a group in your community, ask him or her to explain your needs to the group.

➠ **Ask a social worker, caseworker, or nurse to recommend paid drivers to you.**
Do not try to get paid help on your own. Ask a social worker or nurse involved in the person's care for guidance in finding paid help. They understand the kind of help you need, and they have had experience with different agencies and ways to get help.

➠ **Ask whether the treatment center or medical clinic has its own transportation service.**
Some centers offer free transportation to and from chemotherapy or radiation appointments. These are usually van services, and the person must be prepared to spend half the day at the treatment site. Many enjoy riding with others who are undergoing treatment.

➠ **Use a county medical van or service.**
If treatments are within the county in which the person lives, a county van service may be able to help you. If treatments are in a different county, ask whether the transportation service crosses county lines. The telephone book often has listings for county services at the beginning or end of the book. Look for County Services or, if you live in a larger area, the name of your county.

You can also look on the Internet by searching for your county. Not all counties offer transportation services; call and find out.

Arrange Home Nursing Services, as Necessary

Home nursing services offer care from three types of nursing care professionals: registered nurses, private-duty nurses, and nurses' aides.

➤ Registered nurses

The doctor can prescribe home visits by registered nurses to do skilled nursing procedures and to administer certain chemotherapy medicines at home. A registered nurse can come to the home for short procedures, such as taking blood or urine samples or helping with dressing changes on a wound, ostomy opening, or intravenous (IV) needle site. A registered nurse would also be able to teach the person or a caregiver how to care for an IV line, how to change a dressing on a wound, or how to take or administer medicines correctly. Visits by registered nurses are often short (about an hour), and the cost is covered by insurance once a doctor's approval is received. Registered nurses can also arrange for other care providers to visit, if needed, such as nurses' aides, social workers, speech therapists, occupational therapists, and physical therapists.

Some agencies can send a nurse just to draw blood or perform some other short task. The cost of this visit is seldom covered by insurance, but the fees are usually low. Ask the nurses or social workers to recommend an agency you can call about this service.

Chemotherapy nurses can come to the home when it is difficult to travel to the clinic. These nurses can be the same ones you see at the clinic or doctor's office where chemotherapy is given, or they can be employed by a visiting nurse agency. Ask the clinic nurses or the person's doctor about this possibility.

➤ Private-duty nurses

You can arrange for private-duty nurses without a doctor's approval. Visits from these nurses can last as long as you want; however, many agencies require a minimum visit of four hours. For example, some families find it helpful to arrange for eight hours of overnight care. The cost of this service is usually not covered by insurance, but be sure to ask your insurance carrier to be sure. Private-duty nurses can be registered nurses (called "RNs"), licensed practical nurses (called "LPNs"), or nurses' aides.

➤ Nurses' aides

You can sometimes arrange for nurses' aides for personal care services without a doctor's approval. It is best to check with a social worker, however, to be sure the agency sending the aide is reliable. Nurses' aides can visit to assist you with tasks that do not require a registered nurse. Nurses' aides, also called attendants, can help with bathing, walking, shopping, cooking, and light household chores. Speak with your hospital social worker or contact your American Cancer Society at **800-227-2345** and ask for names and phone numbers of home nursing services near you.

Get Help with Meals and Household Chores, as Necessary

➠ **Call your local Area Agency on Aging or other senior services agency.**
Local Agencies on Aging are good sources of information on services for seniors, from home care to meal delivery. Depending on the community in which you live, there may be other groups. Look in the phone book under senior services or social services, or look online for service organizations in your area. See the section on caregiver resources beginning on page 302. Most cities and small towns have programs that deliver meals to your home, usually through Meals on Wheels. Many of these programs are for senior citizens. If you are under sixty-five, you may still be able to qualify, so call and ask. The cost of the service varies, and you may be eligible for reduced rates. Usually a hot lunch is delivered, along with a cold meal to be eaten later in the day. Meals for special diets are available, including diabetic, low-sodium, and low-fat diets.

➠ **Ask about agencies that help with meal preparation.**
Some agencies have programs where a worker or nurses' aide comes to the home a few times a week and helps by shopping for food and supplies, running errands, preparing meals, and doing light housekeeping.

➠ **Ask church groups or neighbors to organize a small home helper group for meal delivery or chores at your home.**
Many churches are happy to arrange home helpers who can do yard work, window washing, or other chores. Sometimes they arrange for the youth group to get involved.

➠ **Contact your American Cancer Society at 800-227-2345 and ask about groups near you who deliver or help with meals.**

Possible Challenges

Consider the following situations that have been difficult for other caregivers:

"I don't want to ask for help. If people want to help, they'll offer."
Some people feel their friends and relatives should volunteer to help without being asked. If you feel this way, think back to your own experience with ill friends or acquaintances. It can be

difficult sometimes to find the time or inclination to volunteer to help, especially if people are not sure how to help. If people don't volunteer, that doesn't mean they are unwilling or uninterested in helping. Family and friends will probably welcome the opportunity to help if asked because they know they are meeting a specific need.

"No one around here can help drive. They don't have the time or the money for gas. Some don't even have cars, they work, or they are too busy with their families."
You don't know who can help until you ask. Ask other people to help you find drivers. Retirees and people who are temporarily unemployed might have the time to help you solve this problem.

Carrying Out and Adjusting Your Plan

Think about other possible challenges that could interfere with obtaining information about valuable resources in the community. What additional roadblocks could get in the way of following the recommendations in this chapter? Will the person with cancer use the services that are available? How will you explain your needs to the volunteers and staff at community agencies? Develop plans for getting around these challenges using the COPE ideas in the introduction.

Don't wait. Start learning before you need assistance from community agencies and volunteer groups. This valuable information will then be available when you need it.

It often takes time to learn how to make the best use of community agencies and volunteer groups. If you are feeling worn down by your problems, ask someone else to help you work out a solution. Sometimes people who are not directly involved can see new ways to deal with the problem. Talk to a social worker at the hospital or in a social service or health agency. Social workers have a great deal of experience with these problems and can often be creative in helping you get the help you need.

CHAPTER FIVE

Getting Information from Medical Staff

Over the course of the person's illness, you will need a great deal of information to give the best care. Some of this information will be complicated, and often it must come from different sources. It is not surprising that many family caregivers have difficulty getting the information they need. This chapter can help you deal with this problem by describing a sequence of steps to take to obtain medical information.

There are two things to keep in mind with regard to requesting medical information. First, it is usually reasonable to assume the medical staff members want to help you and want to give you the information you need. Second, sometimes staff members will not be allowed to answer your questions, as each medical care organization has its own rules about who can be given information and who is allowed to give that information out. Doctor's offices will have different rules, and hospitals' rules will vary. Even within the same hospital, there are often different rules for the departments caring for inpatients (patients who stay overnight) and outpatients (patients who come and go in the same day), different rules for surgery and oncology, and so on. You will have to identify whom to talk to for information at each new office, department, or hospital.

When to Get Professional Help

If you feel the situation is an emergency and you cannot get the information you need, call the doctor or an emergency room. Be sure the person you talk to understands that you feel this situation is an emergency. Be sure to use the word emergency in your question, and be persistent until you have the information you need.

Remember that you can always ask the American Cancer Society (**800-227-2345** or **cancer.org**) for information. Information on cancer and cancer treatment is available through the Web site or by calling a cancer information specialist through the toll-free number above. Cancer information specialists will listen to your questions and help you find answers, and you may call them as many times as you like. They also know about community services in your area and elsewhere, in case you need to travel for cancer treatments.

What You Can Do

Family caregivers should have all the information they need to provide the best possible care at home. There are five kinds of information usually needed:

- an understanding of the condition—What is it? What causes it? What can family caregivers expect to accomplish in dealing with the condition?
- what to do to deal with and prevent the condition
- challenges that might interfere
- how to carry out and monitor your plan
- when to call for professional help

You will need all of this information if you are to meet your caregiving responsibilities. Feel free to ask for information and persist until you have it. Your goal is to get the medical information you need as quickly and efficiently as possible and with as little stress as possible for both you and the medical staff. Doing three things can improve your ability to get the information you need quickly and efficiently:

- **Phrase your questions clearly.**
- **Learn which people to ask.**
- **Ask the person with cancer to get the needed information.**

Phrase Your Questions Clearly

Know exactly what information you need, and state your questions clearly:

➠ **Ask yourself, "What do I need to know to do my job as a home caregiver?"**
This question is one of the best ways to begin deciding what information you need. This question focuses your attention on what is most important; otherwise, you may find yourself asking a lot of questions without finding out what you really need to know.

➠ **When you ask questions, first say what you need to know and then why you need to know it.**
It is easier for someone else to understand your question if you start with a clear statement of the information you need. Then you can tell him or her why you need to know and the listener will understand the reasoning behind what you are saying. For example, let's assume that the person you are caring for had malaria when he was in the service. You notice that some of his symptoms

after chemotherapy are similar to malaria, and these symptoms make you worried that the malaria is returning. When you ask your question, start by asking if the symptoms could be due to malaria. Then explain the reason you are concerned: he had malaria when he was in the service, and the symptoms after chemotherapy are very similar. The listener then knows both what you want to know and why.

IIIII➡ Write out your questions, and check them with other people.

Keep a list of questions you want to ask at the next doctor visit or home health nurse visit. Writing down your questions beforehand is one of the best ways to be sure you are being clear. Having a nurse or social worker read your list before you see the doctor is a good way to check on your clarity. If you get flustered at the visit, which happens to many people, then you can read your questions from your list.

Learn Which People to Ask

Different people can give you different kinds of information, and the contact person can vary with different doctors, hospitals, and clinics. You need to know who can give you the information you need for each new treatment setting. The following suggestions can help:

IIIII➡ Learn which staff members give out which types of information.

The best way to find this out is to ask a medical staff person, such as a nurse, social worker, or doctor. Nurses or social workers are usually good resources. Start your question with "Who can tell me . . . ?" Try, for example, "Who can tell me when my husband will be discharged?" or "Who can tell me when my mother's treatments are scheduled?" See the list on the next page of the types of information that different health care professionals can usually give you.

IIIII➡ Be prepared to learn the rules for every new group of health care staff that you encounter.

It is a good idea to ask questions early on, as soon as you begin working with a new treatment team. You can avoid problems later by using this approach.

IIIII➡ Be persistent!

Pleasant persistence almost always pays off. If medical staff members say they don't know or can't tell you, ask who can. You may have to ask several people. Medical care can be complicated, which means that getting medical information can be complicated, too. Don't get discouraged, and don't be afraid to ask follow-up questions until you are very clear about the answers you received. You have a right to the information you need to be the best possible caregiver. Getting information will become easier as you gain a better understanding of the medical care system.

▐▶ **Ask a nurse, social worker, or other member of the health care team to get the information you need.**

Sometimes the health care professional with whom you need to talk is not available when you need the information or does not provide the specific information you need. If any of these things happen, a good strategy is to ask a nurse or social worker to get information for you. Nurses and social workers understand medical terminology and how medical organizations work. They are also usually good at explaining this information to patients and their caregivers. Choose nurses or social workers with whom you feel comfortable, and tell them what information you need and why you can't get it yourself. Then ask for their help.

Sources of information

Different medical professionals can usually provide different kinds of health care information:

Physicians

Physicians know about treatment plans, the prognosis (the likelihood of cure or remission and the usual course of the disease), how often the person—for example, your husband—will be evaluated, how often he needs to see a doctor, when he should be admitted to a hospital, what medicines should be taken and when, results of tests, and whether the treatment is working.

Nurses

Nurses know about the management of side effects of treatments, appointment schedules, nutrition information, results of some tests (this depends on the doctor or hospital policies), and how and when to take medications.

Social workers

Social workers help in dealing with family and emotional problems, arranging for medical care at home, admitting the person to a nursing home or hospice program, getting financial help, and determining whether the person with cancer qualifies for government programs.

Use this list as a starting point for getting information, but be prepared for lots of exceptions. Hospital physicians have different titles, such as attending, fellow, resident, hospitalist, and consultant. They may also be identified by their professional specialty title, such as surgeon, oncologist, radiation oncologist, pathologist, and so on. Depending on your medical needs, doctors with different titles and specialties have different responsibilities and can give you different kinds of information. When several physicians are involved, one member of the team will be coordinating the care and will be known as the coordinating physician.

Ask the Person with Cancer to Get the Needed Information

The person with cancer sees all the people on the health care team more frequently or regularly and can be helpful in getting information that you need as a caregiver. Remember, though, that he or she may have other things on his or her mind or be tired when he or she sees the health care team. To help prevent questions from going unanswered, you may want to write down your questions. You may also want to ask one of the staff (such as a nurse or social worker) to remind the person with cancer to ask the questions and to assist that person with writing down the answers, if necessary. Sometimes the person with cancer may not want to ask certain questions because the answers may be upsetting. In this case, respect the person's wishes and try to speak to the doctor or nurse in private.

Possible Challenges

Consider the following situations that have been difficult for other caregivers:

"My questions are stupid."

No questions are stupid. You and the medical staff want to give the best possible care to the person with cancer. To provide quality care, you need to know what to do and why it needs to be done. It is the medical staff's job to answer your questions and to help educate you.

"I feel confused by the health care system."

Medical staff use unfamiliar words, have peculiar titles, and are organized into groups with unfamiliar names. It is not surprising that so many people are confused by medical environments. It can be almost as confusing as going to a foreign country. Many people, when they travel to a foreign county, get a guide who speaks the language. You can use this model for learning about the health care system. Your guides can be health care staff, such as nurses and social workers, who know the system. Ask them to explain the system to you: what titles mean, what different groups do, and what medical terms mean. As you learn about the system, you will soon be using medical terms yourself and finding your way around like a veteran.

"I feel intimidated by medical staff."

Some people feel that health care professionals are so important or busy that their time should not be taken up with questions. Do not be intimidated. Ask your questions. The doctors and other medical staff are there to help people. To provide proper care, the staff must give caregivers the information they need to care for the person with cancer at home.

"If I need to know something, the doctor will tell me."

Although the doctor will try to tell you everything you need to know, he or she can't always remember what you were told on previous occasions, may assume that someone else told you, or may simply forget to tell you certain things. Tell the doctor what information you need and make sure all your questions are answered.

"If I ask too many questions, the staff will think I'm a nuisance, and then they won't take good care of the person I'm helping."

It is unlikely that the staff will think you are a nuisance. However, even if they do, their opinions will not affect how they treat the person with cancer. Medical professionals are trained to treat everyone to the best of their ability, no matter what opinions they have about the person. To do otherwise is malpractice.

Carrying Out and Adjusting Your Plan

Think of other challenges that could interfere with carrying out your plan to obtain more information. What additional roadblocks could get in the way of following the recommendations in this chapter? Will the medical staff cooperate? Will other people help you locate the necessary sources of information? How will you explain your needs to medical staff? Develop plans for getting around these challenges using the COPE ideas outlined in the introduction.

Ask questions. The more questions you ask, the easier it will become. In the beginning, you may want to write your questions down and read them out loud. Practice beforehand what you will say. Set deadlines for getting certain information.

Keep track of the number of times you have problems getting information you need. If you believe medical staff are not giving you the information you need, consider making an appointment with the doctor who is responsible for the person's care. At the appointment, ask him or her your questions. Explain the problems you have had in getting information, and ask how to avoid these problems in the future. Note that you will most likely be charged for this appointment, since many insurers will not pay for such appointments. Ask about costs when making the appointment. If you cannot afford to pay, you can ask to have the fee waived, or you can ask if your meeting can be scheduled as part of the person's regular meeting with the physician. When you speak with the doctor, don't be angry and don't be intimidated. Being angry only makes the other person angry, too, and if you are intimidated it will be more difficult to explain the situation clearly. A calm, objective approach works best.

Most hospitals have patient advocates or similar staff members. These people are knowledgeable about how to deal with problems you may have with the hospital. They can help you get necessary information, and they may be able to change the way some things in the hospital are handled. You may help future patients by telling patient advocates about problems you are having.

As a last resort, the person with cancer always has the right to change doctors or treatment settings. If he or she is considering a change, be sure the new setting will provide the support you need.

CHAPTER SIX

Finances and Caregiving

Cancer treatment can be very expensive. For some people, cancer treatment can ultimately lead to financial problems. As a caregiver, you may already be responsible for the family's finances or you may assume that responsibility while the person is undergoing treatment. Whether you are new to this task or experienced at managing money, the complexities of paying for cancer treatment can be overwhelming. You can avoid some financial problems through organization and good management of the family's finances. This will include understanding the person's insurance benefits, knowing about and exploring other sources of financial assistance, keeping sound records, and making a financial plan.

It is important to discuss financial matters early and develop a plan. Likewise, it is important to deal with any financial *problems* early—before they become crises. If problems arise, try to address them as soon as you can. If you owe money, talking to the creditor or institution early makes it more likely that they will be willing to work with you. Many financial problems can be averted or lessened by taking steps to manage the finances of cancer treatment and addressing problems quickly.

When to Get Professional Help

Talk with your hospital social worker or financial counselor early. Most hospitals have social workers on staff that can assist you with finding resources in your area and helping you identify your options. Social workers are usually the best source of information about how to get help with medical expenses and how best to deal with insurers. Do not wait until you are having problems to talk with someone about resources and options. Discussing financial issues early, and often, can help prevent problems later on.

What You Can Do

There are a number of ways the caregiver can help to manage the financial aspects of cancer and cancer treatment:

- **Learn about the person's benefits.**
- **Manage insurance issues.**
- **Learn about other sources of financial assistance.**
- **Keep thorough records.**
- **Make a financial plan.**

Learn About the Person's Benefits

Understanding the benefits for which the person is eligible is essential to developing a sound financial plan. Questions about insurance coverage will almost inevitably arise at some point during the person's cancer treatment. There are many different types of health insurance and health service plans. It is very important to understand what type of plan the person has and what kinds of expenses the plan covers. The person may have a private health insurance plan, a government-funded health plan, a combination, or may be uninsured. Even if the person has health insurance, you may find that the expenses associated with cancer treatment may not all be covered or may not be covered in full. Costs will vary depending on the type of treatment prescribed. The cost of chemotherapy, for example, can vary greatly depending on the drugs used, the dosages, and the frequency and duration of treatments. The types of treatments that are covered may vary between insurers. If the person does not have health insurance, there may be other sources of financial assistance available. These options are discussed further beginning on page 62.

Manage Insurance Issues

DO NOT allow health insurance to expire. Even if the person is switching from one plan to another, do not let the first policy lapse until the new policy has gone into effect.

▥➤ **Find out the details of the individual insurance plan and its coverage.**
Contact a customer service representative with the insurance provider to ask detailed questions about the policy and what expenses are and are not covered. Get a copy of the plan's summary description (SPD), which tells you how the plan works, what benefits it provides, and how to get the benefits or file a claim. If you think the person might need more insurance, ask the insurance carrier if it is available.

▥➤ **Before the person begins treatment, find out whether the prescribed treatment will be covered under the person's insurance policy.**

This information can help the person make informed decisions before beginning treatment.

▥➤ **Talk to a caseworker or financial assistance planner in the hospital or doctor's office.**
This person may be able to help you fill out claims for insurance coverage or reimbursement and help guide you through this process. Often, companies or hospitals can work with you to make special payment arrangements if you let them know about your situation.

▥➤ **Submit claims for all medical expenses even when you are not sure whether they are covered.**

▥➤ **Keep accurate and complete records of claims submitted, pending, and paid, as well as copies of all paperwork related to claims.**
These may include letters of medical necessity, explanations of benefits, bills, receipts, requests for sick leave or family medical leave (FMLA), and correspondence with insurance companies.

▥➤ **Send in bills for reimbursement as soon as they are received.**
If you become overwhelmed with bills, get help. Talk with the hospital social worker or call the American Cancer Society at **800-227-2345**.

▥➤ **When dealing with insurance-related questions that come up over the course of the person's treatment, follow these guidelines:**
- Talk to a customer service representative with the health insurance provider or the hospital's social worker or financial counselor for help.
- Contact the consumer advocacy office of the government agency that oversees the insurance provider. You can find your state's insurance commissioner in the blue pages of your phone book or visit the National Association of Insurance Commissioners on the Web at http://naic.org/state_web_map.htm.
- Learn about the laws pertaining to health insurance that protect the public. The Agency for Healthcare Research and Quality provides information on health insurance on the Web at www.ahrq.gov/consumer/insurancega/.

▥➤ **If a claim is denied or a prescribed service is refused, follow up with the insurance provider.**
At some point during the person's treatment, you may be notified that an insurance claim has been denied or that the insurance company will not cover a certain test, procedure, or service that has been prescribed by the doctor. If this happens, you have the option to resubmit the claim

for consideration or to appeal the insurance company's decision. In this situation, it is important to work closely with the customer service representative or case manager at the insurance company to resolve the matter. Follow these guidelines when appealing a denied claim:

- Review the insurance policy again to ensure you understand the specific benefits provided by the plan.
- Contact the insurer and request a full explanation in writing of why the claim was denied.
- Contact the doctor's office and request a written explanation of the prescribed service and justification as to why it is necessary. Provide a copy of this information to the insurer and keep a copy for your records.
- Resubmit the claim with the documentation provided by the doctor.
- Ask to speak with a case manager or supervisor at the insurance company who may have the authority to reverse the decision.
- Be persistent when seeking a resolution.

Learn About Other Sources of Financial Assistance

If the person does not have private health insurance, he or she may be eligible for government-funded health care programs or other assistance provided to people without insurance. Many people are eligible for financial assistance but do not know it. Social workers are usually the best source of information about how to get help with medical expenses, and they can help you determine whether the person with cancer qualifies for assistance.

⯈ Medicare and Medicaid

Medicare is a federal program funded through the Social Security System. It provides health insurance for people who are at least sixty-five years old, people who are permanently disabled and receive disability benefits from Social Security, or people who have permanent kidney failure treated with dialysis or a transplant. For questions about Medicare, call 800-MEDICARE (800-633-4227).

Medicaid is a joint federal-state government program that provides medical care for individuals and families with low incomes and limited resources. Contact your state Medicaid office to find out whether the person with cancer is eligible for Medicaid and whether the recommended therapy is covered. To learn more about Medicare and Medicaid, visit the U.S. Department of Health and Human Services on the Web at www.cms.hhs.gov. Not all health care providers accept Medicare and Medicaid, so it is important to check with your health care provider before services are rendered.

⫸ Veteran's benefits

If the person has ever been on active duty in the military, he or she may qualify for benefits through the Department of Veteran Affairs. Several factors determine eligibility, including length of service, the type of discharge received, disability, income, and availability of services in the area. The number of veteran's medical facilities has recently declined, and benefits for veterans can change often. Call 800-827-1000 or visit www.va.gov/healtheligibility/ for the most up-to-date information.

⫸ Hill-Burton Program

The Hill-Burton Program is a federal program that provides free or reduced-cost medical care to qualified individuals through approximately two hundred health care facilities nationwide. Each facility chooses which services it will provide for free or at a reduced cost. Eligibility is based on income and family size. To locate a Hill-Burton facility, visit the Web site of the Health Resources and Services Administration at http://www.hrsa.gov/hillburton/hillburtonfacilities.htm or call the Hill-Burton Hotline at 800-638-0742.

⫸ Social Security

If the person with cancer becomes disabled during treatment, he or she may qualify to receive Supplemental Security Income or Social Security Disability Income through the Social Security Administration. The applicant must meet a very narrow definition of disability according to the Social Security Administration to qualify for either program. Call 800-772-1213 or visit www.socialsecurity.gov to find out more.

⫸ Pharmaceutical patient assistance programs

Some drug companies offer patient assistance programs that provide discounted or free medicines to people who do not qualify for other assistance. Additional benefits may include insurance reimbursement and referrals to copay relief programs. The programs and services offered may differ for each company. Contact the drug company that makes the person's medication to find out whether the person qualifies for any available programs. You can also talk to the hospital's social worker or doctor or contact the Partnership for Prescription Assistance at 888-477-2669 or on the Web at www.pparx.org to learn more about available programs.

⫸ Nonprofit programs

A number of nonprofit organizations provide financial assistance for medical expenses associated with cancer treatment, as well as practical needs such as transportation, child care, and domestic help. Each organization has eligibility criteria and may only provide assistance for people with certain types of cancer. Some community-based groups and religious organizations offer assistance to people who have been affected by illness. Talk to community organizations or local churches about your needs. You may also choose to speak with a social worker through the hospital, or contact the American Cancer Society at **800-227-2345** or **cancer.org** to locate more financial resources in your area.

Keep Thorough Records

Keep careful records of medical bills, insurance claims, and other health care–related correspondence. This will make managing treatment costs much easier and will also help prevent problems down the road. Organized financial records will also be useful if you have to demonstrate the need for financial assistance. Here are some tips to help with record keeping:

▶ **Set up a filing system exclusively for health care–related paperwork.**
Use a file cabinet, binder, or expanding folder to store important paperwork. Save all bills, benefits statements, payment receipts, and cancelled checks.

▶ **Determine who is responsible for what.**
Make sure to find out from the doctor's office or hospital whether office staff will be filing insurance claims on the person's behalf or whether you are responsible for paying for services and submitting claims to the insurance provider for reimbursement.

▶ **Review each bill and benefits statement carefully and check to make sure they are correct.**
Make notes about any questionable charges or claim denials. Follow up immediately with your insurer to resolve any disputes.

▶ **Work closely with the staff member who handles billing for each provider so that you can be sure of what is owed to each provider.**
Because of the complicated method of billing used by many hospitals and health care providers, it can sometimes be difficult to determine what is owed to whom.

▶ **Keep track of all out-of-pocket medical expenses that are not covered by insurance.**
These expenses may be deductible from the person's income taxes.

Make a Financial Plan

Planning ahead for the anticipated expenses of cancer treatment can not only help prevent financial crises, but it can also help you feel more in control of the situation. Consider the following approach when making a financial plan:

⫸ Collect the facts.

Talk to the doctor about what to expect during cancer treatment so you can plan accordingly. How long will the person need to be out of work? How many medical procedures are anticipated? How long will prescription medicines be needed? Some decisions about the person's treatment might be hard to anticipate, but thinking about the financial worse-case scenario could help you be prepared for unanticipated expenses that may occur down the road.

⫸ Calculate the expenses.

Collect as much information as possible about the expenses you expect to be associated with the person's cancer treatment. Make sure to consider the following expenses:

- travel costs (including gasoline and parking)
- lodging (if treatment is done far from home)
- meals during travel or clinic visits
- hospital stays
- out-of-pocket medical expenses
- prescription drug costs
- home health care costs
- special equipment, clothing, or nutritional supplements
- services such as childcare, housekeeping, and meal preparation

⫸ Calculate your financial resources.

Collect as much information as possible about the financial resources available. What is the total household income? This information is often used to calculate eligibility for financial assistance. What portion of the medical bills will the insurance provider cover? Does the person with cancer qualify for any financial assistance? Does financial assistance cover the prescribed treatments? How much money is available in savings? What other assets are available, including property, real estate, and investments? Are viaticals or living benefits appropriate for the person with cancer? (Read more about viaticals and living benefits on the next page.) Answers to these questions will help form a picture of the total financial resources available.

Once you have collected as much information as possible and calculated your expenses and available financial resources, you can work toward making a plan to pay for cancer treatment. You may be able to pay bills in installments to make the payments more manageable. Contact the financial counselor or business credit office at your doctor's office or treatment center to find out whether staff can help you set up a payment plan. Some hospitals, doctors, and pharmacies are willing to submit bills to the insurance company and bill you only for what the insurance company does not pay. This prevents you from having to pay the entire bill up front and wait for reimbursement from the insurance company.

VIATICALS AND LIVING BENEFITS

A viatical settlement is the sale of an existing life insurance policy before the policy matures. The payout for a viatical is often 60 to 80 percent of the face value of the life insurance policy. It may also be tax-free. Most insurance companies that buy viatical settlements will only buy policies from people with terminal illnesses whose life expectancy has been certified by a doctor. The insurance company becomes the new owner of the policy, pays all premiums, and will be the beneficiary when the original policy holder dies. This transaction may be an option for some people who are experiencing financial difficulty. It is important, however, to weigh this decision carefully: once the policy is sold, the transaction is usually not reversible.

Most life insurance policies are payable after the policy owner dies. In some cases, however, insurance companies make it possible for beneficiaries to collect all or part of the death benefits before the policy owner dies. These are called "living benefits" or "accelerated benefits." Living benefits can range from 25 percent to 95 percent of the death benefit and can be used to cover expenses associated with cancer treatment. The amount of living benefits paid will depend on many factors, including the policy's face value, the terms of the contract, and the state in which the policy owner lives. Before making a viatical settlement or living benefits part of your financial plan, contact the insurance company to obtain a quote and additional details about its requirements for those steps.

Carrying Out and Adjusting the Plan

Make sure to seek out all available resources to help and deal with any financial problems early, when they can be resolved more easily. Start using the ideas in this chapter early. Don't wait until you feel overwhelmed.

The financial costs associated with cancer treatment can be overwhelming. Caregivers can be instrumental to managing the family's finances while the person with cancer is undergoing treatment. For more information about dealing with the financial aspects of cancer treatment, consult the resource guide beginning on page 299, or contact the American Cancer Society at **800-227-2345** or **cancer.org**.

Part II

Emotional Responses to Cancer and Cancer Treatment

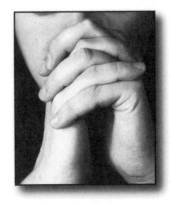

THIS SECTION CAN HELP YOU DEAL WITH EMOTIONAL RESPONSES TO CANCER, such as anxiety and depression, whether they are affecting you or the person with cancer. It explains the feelings experienced by many caregivers and people with cancer. Encourage your loved one to read these chapters, and then you can work together as a team.

Unlike the physical side effects discussed in parts III and IV, depression and anxiety can affect the person with cancer and the caregiver or other family members. A cancer diagnosis can be a source of stress for the whole family, and the responsibilities of caregiving can make it difficult for some people to cope.

Some people, when faced with a cancer diagnosis, act as if nothing has happened and deny that there is anything to worry about. This reaction can upset family members, and it also can be a barrier to expressing feelings or practical concerns. Ignoring the fact that one has cancer can become a serious problem if the person refuses treatment or does things that interfere with treatment. It can also be a problem if loved ones feel overly constricted in talking with the person with cancer and in what they say or do around him or her. Another possible problem in ignoring a cancer diagnosis is that important personal decisions may be neglected.

Sometimes family members or close friends wish that the person with cancer would be more open and willing to express feelings. This process may be difficult for the person with cancer, and family members will have to be sensitive and creative in their approach. Sometimes even ideas that seem silly at first can turn out to be useful. In the introduction, we discussed brainstorming as part of the COPE approach to problem solving. Brainstorming is a good way to think of new and unusual solutions to problems. Other people have found these approaches helpful in encouraging conversations about feelings:

- The person talks about his or her feelings to a trusted person outside the family (such as a friend or clergy member), who then expresses them to the family.
- The family and the person with cancer express their feelings by letter or e-mail.
- The person with cancer and the family set aside thirty minutes once a week for a session in which they agree to talk about how everyone is feeling.
- Family members write down the feelings they want to discuss and give the person the option of answering only certain ones.

These examples may not fit your situation, but they have been helpful to others and show that being open to new and creative ideas can help to resolve difficult problems. If, despite your or others' best efforts, the person with cancer still can't be more open about feelings, it is usually best to let the person use coping strategies that have worked in the past rather than expecting him or her to change.

This section and the two that follow are primarily organized to help you deal with problems or side effects that may come up during cancer treatment and caregiving. Each chapter is organized under five major topics:

1. Understanding the condition
   - when the problem will likely occur
   - what kinds of things can be done to help
   - what goals to have when dealing with the condition

2. When to get professional help
   - when to call for help immediately
   - when to call during office hours
   - what information to have ready when you're calling

3. What you can do
   - what you can do to manage the problem at home
   - what you can do to help to prevent the problem

4. Possible challenges
   - recognizing problems
   - how to deal with problems you may have in carrying out your plans

5. Carrying out and adjusting the plan
   - how to monitor progress
   - how quickly to expect change
   - what to do if the plan isn't working

The information in this section fits most situations, but your situation may be different. If the person's doctor or nurse provides different instructions, always follow the advice of your health care providers. For more information on emotional conditions and coping with cancer and cancer treatment, contact your American Cancer Society at **800-227-2345** or visit the Web site at **cancer.org**.

CHAPTER SEVEN

Anxiety

During a stressful illness such as cancer, it is normal to feel anxious, whether you are the person with cancer or the caregiver. Medical procedures or fear of the future can cause anxiety. Caregivers may worry about the person's illness and their own ability to cope with caregiving. Sometimes the anxiety of the person with cancer makes caregivers anxious. Poor communication between the person with cancer and family and friends can be a source of anxiety for everyone.

Almost everyone with cancer feels nervous at some time during treatment. This feeling is normal and natural. As a caregiver, you can help during periods of nervousness by being supportive and understanding. Let the person know that you understand why he or she feels nervous. Be available to listen and encourage him or her. Following familiar routines can also reduce nervousness. As treatment gets under way, familiarity with the medical staff's routines can help. Friendly and supportive medical staff can also help a great deal in reducing a person's nervousness.

What Is Anxiety?

Nervous or anxious feelings are a normal response to stressful situations, and nervousness is very common among people undergoing cancer treatment. Everyone has felt anxious at various times in life. For example, people often feel anxious or nervous before a job interview, before talking to a group of people, or when they are worried about someone they love. Such nervous tension can sometimes help people. For example, many actors say that they have "butterflies in their stomach," or anxious moments, before they perform. Sometimes people actually enjoy feelings of anxiety, like when they are watching a horse race or riding a roller coaster.

When people become so nervous that it is constant and interferes with their quality of life and their ability to cope, we call this anxiety. People experience anxiety in many different ways:

- nervousness
- tension
- panicky feelings
- confusion
- fear
- feeling something bad is going to happen
- feelings of losing control
- anger or irritation

A person experiencing nervousness or anxiety may also have the following physical symptoms:

- sweaty palms
- upset stomach
- tight feelings in the stomach
- shaking or tremors
- difficulty breathing
- racing pulse
- hot and flushed face
- diarrhea or constipation
- frequent urination
- headaches

Sometimes these feelings come and go fairly quickly. Other times these feelings last a long time.

When anxious feelings are very strong and are dominated by fear, they can interfere with everyday living. When they last a long time—more than a week, for example—they can prevent people from doing things that are important to them. Learning effective coping strategies can help keep anxiety from disrupting your quality of life.

One of the difficult things about anxiety is that people may not recognize that they are experiencing it. They may think that they are just worried, even as anxiety symptoms become more severe. Family and friends of the person with cancer can help by being alert to signs of anxiety in the person, pointing out anxiety if they see it, and helping the person control anxiety before it gets severe.

Anxiety Related to Cancer

A cancer diagnosis often causes some anxious feelings. Some people feel afraid, nervous, or overwhelmed. Others may feel panicky, as if they have lost control of their lives. These reactions are normal and may last from a few days to a few weeks.

Many people with cancer experience some anxiety during their treatments. Anxiety can be caused by the following triggers:

- fear of being a burden to family and friends
- fear of getting sicker and having a shorter life
- pain and discomfort or fear of pain and discomfort
- medicines used to treat cancer
- worries about medical procedures

Anxiety can make physical symptoms more intense. For example, a person who is in pain usually reports more severe pain when he or she is experiencing anxious feelings. Although some nervousness is normal for people with cancer, it can become so severe that it interferes with their ability to cope with the illness. Anxiety may make some people reluctant to visit the doctor and may even make them think of dropping out of treatment. Severe anxiety can also seriously reduce the quality of life of people with cancer.

Controlling anxiety is primarily in the hands of the person experiencing it. As the caregiver, you can give encouragement and help. Try not to feel guilty if, in spite of your best efforts, the person with cancer is very anxious. If the anxiety is severe, a professional may be needed who can use special techniques such as anti-anxiety medicines or stress management techniques.

When to Get Professional Help

Speak with the doctor, nurse, psychologist, or social worker if any of the following conditions exist:

- ***The person seriously considers stopping treatment.*** Sometimes people skip treatments or avoid visits to the doctor because of anxiety.
- ***The person has a history of severe anxiety requiring professional help or therapy.*** It is important for the health care team to know about any past problems with anxiety.
- ***Anxiety has seriously lowered quality of life.*** Professional help is needed if anxiety symptoms are interfering with daily activities or are upsetting to the person with cancer.
- ***Anxiety is increasingly dominating all aspects of care.*** Some people are hesitant to ask for help with emotional problems. They need to understand that being upset during a major illness is normal, as is seeking help for these problems.

Call the doctor, nurse, or social worker if any of the following symptoms persist for several days:

- severe problems with sleeping
- feelings of dread and serious apprehension

- trembling, twitching, and feeling shaky
- fluttering stomach with nausea and diarrhea
- increased heart rate or feeling a rapid pulse
- wide mood swings that cannot be controlled
- shortness of breath

Some of these symptoms could be caused by cancer or side effects of the treatments, as well as by anxiety. The doctor treating the person can evaluate the causes of these symptoms. It is best to start with the person's oncologist or family physician, who will be familiar with the person and the treatments he or she is receiving. Ask for an evaluation of possible causes of the anxiety and recommendations for treatment or referral. A doctor can evaluate whether a change in treatment is needed or whether anti-anxiety medicines could help the person. Be alert to whether family members also need help for anxiety. Physicians can also make referrals to mental health professionals, including psychologists, psychiatrists, social workers, and nurse counselors. If you are not sure whether professional help is needed, ask a nurse or social worker for guidance.

What You Can Do

Don't expect to eliminate all anxiety. Some anxiety is both normal and understandable. You can, however, help keep anxiety from becoming severe or seriously interfering with the person's quality of life or medical treatments. You can help the person manage anxiety by encouraging him or her to follow these guidelines:

- **Identify the causes of the anxiety.**
- **Talk with someone who has been through a similar situation.**
- **Engage in pleasant, distracting activities.**
- **Use relaxation techniques.**

Identify the Causes of the Anxiety

Understanding what is causing the anxiety is key to controlling it.

▥➡ **Identify what thoughts are causing the anxiety.**

Anxiety has two parts: thoughts and feelings. Worried thoughts lead to nervous feelings, which lead to additional worried thoughts, and so on. To stop this cycle, you must first determine what thoughts are causing the anxiety and why. For example, if going into the hospital is upsetting, ask what makes the hospital upsetting. Perhaps the anxiety is fueled by a fear of being left alone or concern about paying hospital bills. Sometimes you won't be able to find an exact cause of the anxiety. Professional help may be useful in this situation.

74

▸ **If the person is anxious about medical procedures, identify what is upsetting about the procedure.**

Is it needles, pain, being alone, being naked, being in an enclosed space? If the person cannot explain what makes the procedure upsetting, ask him or her: "How would you change this procedure so it wouldn't upset you?"

▸ **If the person is anxious about hearing news from the health care team, try to find out what kind of news the person is afraid of hearing.**

Is it being told more treatments are required? Having to be admitted to the hospital? The prospect of being unable to do certain things in the future? It is important to be tactful and sensitive when asking these types of questions. Just talking about a stressful event may make the person more anxious. Pay close attention to what the person is saying and do not interrupt. It may be helpful to repeat back what you've heard to be sure you understand. Listening to someone who is experiencing anxiety can itself be helpful by showing the person that someone understands his or her feelings. It also allows the person to talk about the problem, which can help put it in perspective.

▸ **Get the exact facts.**

Information can help reduce anxiety. For example, if the person is worried that the doctor will say the disease has worsened, find out when the doctor will be able to assess how well the treatment is working. You may find out that the doctor will not know whether the cancer is responding to treatment for another eight weeks. If needles are upsetting to the person, try to find out details about tests beforehand so that unnecessary anxiety can be eliminated.

▸ **Look for ways around the problem.**

When you have information about the situation, you may find there are ways to get around a problem that is causing anxiety. For example, if having blood drawn causes anxiety, find out whether blood could be drawn with a small prick on the finger. If the person is worried about being alone during a procedure, ask if you can be with him or her during that time.

Talk with Someone Who Has Been Through a Similar Situation

It is often reassuring to hear about what happened to someone else and how that person reacted during a stressful experience. It can be helpful to know that someone else got through this experience and can help to reduce feelings of isolation. This reassurance can make the future seem more manageable, even if the experience was difficult for the other person.

Choose this person carefully; some people can be more reassuring than others. In general, though, most people find talking to someone who has been through a similar experience reduces worry and anxiety. Most people who have been through scary experiences are happy to talk to others about them. The treatment team may be able to refer you to a support group for people who have gone through similar experiences.

Engage in Pleasant, Distracting Activities

Helping the person with cancer relax and enjoy pleasant activities can help reduce anxiety. There are many types of enjoyable activities that can be helpful to a person who is anxious. Spending time with other people, tasks that provide a sense of accomplishment, and activities that distract from thoughts of the anxiety-causing situation can all be beneficial.

⫸ **Increase companionship and time spent with friends and family.**
Being with people the person enjoys is an excellent way to take attention away from what is causing the anxiety. It can also give family and friends the opportunity to express their love and concern for the person. Knowing that other people care and are available to help gives people strength and confidence in facing frightening experiences.

Use Relaxation Techniques

Encourage the person with cancer to use relaxation techniques. Relaxation is a skill that can be used to counteract anxiety. You cannot be anxious and relaxed at the same time. When you do things that make the person with cancer feel relaxed, anxiety decreases.

There are many ways to feel more relaxed. Prayer or meditation helps many people when they are in tense situations. Many people find certain kinds of music relaxing. Walking or mild exercise can also reduce anxiety, and repetitive deep breathing helps some people to relax their minds and bodies. You can also purchase guided relaxation exercises as audio recordings, which teach relaxation as a skill. The exercise below gives an example of a common type of relaxation technique.

Do this exercise regularly—once a day is best. Try not to do the exercise within an hour after eating, since digestion can interfere with the body's ability to relax certain muscles. Practice this exercise when you are not feeling rushed. In the beginning, it may help to have someone else read you the instructions. You can also record the instructions and play them during the exercise. When practicing, choose a time when you will not be disturbed. Tell the other people in your household what you are doing and ask them to be quiet.

1. Sit quietly in a comfortable position (such as in an easy chair or on the sofa).
2. Close your eyes.
3. Deeply relax your muscles, beginning with your face and working your way down your entire body (neck, shoulders, chest, arms, hands, stomach, legs) and ending with your feet. Imagine the tension flowing out through your feet.

4. Concentrate your attention on your head, and relax your head even further by thinking, "I'm going to let all the tension flow out of my head. I'm letting go of the tension, and I'm letting warm feelings of relaxation smooth out the muscles in my head and face. I'm becoming more relaxed." Repeat these steps for each part of your body: neck, shoulders, arms, hands, chest, abdomen, legs, and feet. Do this slowly—spend enough time to feel more relaxed before going on to the next part of the body.

5. When your body feels very relaxed, concentrate on your breathing. Breathe slowly and deeply through your nose. Pay attention to your breathing. Slowly breathe in. As you breathe out, say the word calm silently to yourself. Repeat this step with every breath. It can help you relax more if you concentrate on the word calm. Continue breathing deeply, becoming more and more relaxed.

6. Continue this exercise for ten to fifteen minutes. Remain relaxed and breathe slowly. At the end of the exercise, slowly open your eyes to become adjusted to the light in the room, and sit quietly for a few minutes.

When the exercise is over, think about how you feel and whether you had any problems relaxing. One problem can be drifting and distracting thoughts. If you find your thoughts drifting the next time you practice, think to yourself, "Let relaxation happen at its own pace." If a distracting thought occurs, let it pass. Let it fly away like a bird. Don't fight it. Concentrate more on the word calm. Let the thought drift by and repeat the word calm over and over again as your breathing gets slower and deeper and you become more and more relaxed.

After you become skilled at this exercise, you will find it is easy to apply these skills when you are getting tense. With practice, people can learn to consciously relax their muscles. They can then learn to use this skill when they are in tense situations.

For example, if you are feeling tense while waiting to see the doctor or waiting for treatment to begin, you can easily close your eyes for a few minutes and use this exercise to relax and feel calm.

It's a good idea to learn relaxation techniques early in the cancer experience—before anxiety becomes severe. These coping skills may keep severe anxiety from happening.

Possible Challenges

Consider the following situations that have been difficult for other caregivers:

"My problems are real. I have to face them even if they make me anxious."

Agree that the problems are real. A certain amount of anxiety about them is normal and understandable; however, research and experience show that severe anxiety interferes with the ability to solve problems. Managing anxiety makes problem solving easier.

"I can't stop the thoughts that make me anxious. They keep coming back and racing around my head."

It's scary to feel like you can't control your thoughts. It may be useful to try some techniques that may reduce anxious thoughts and even stop them. In the chapter on depression, there is a section on stopping negative thoughts. These techniques can also work for anxiety.

"Because I'm the caregiver, I feel like I have to help everyone else with problems. I'm always tired, and I'm becoming frustrated."

Spending a lot of time with someone who is very anxious can be stressful and can also make you anxious. You need to take time for yourself—to deal with your own problems. Use ideas in this chapter and the chapter on depression to care for yourself, as well as for the person with cancer. Try to involve as many people as possible in carrying out this plan. More support will help both of you.

Carrying Out and Adjusting Your Plan

Think of other challenges that could interfere with your plan to manage anxiety. What additional roadblocks could get in the way of following the recommendations in this chapter? Will the person with cancer cooperate? Will other people help? How will you explain your needs to other people? Do you have the time and energy to carry out the plan? Develop plans for getting around these roadblocks by using the COPE ideas discussed in the introduction.

Your first step is to talk about anxiety with the person with cancer. You are a team. You need to agree on how you will manage anxiety together. If you think anxiety is likely at certain times, make plans for what to do at these times to minimize or prevent anxiety. It is always easier to help someone manage anxiety before it becomes serious or overwhelming.

Stay alert to the possibility that professional help may be needed. Review the section "When to Get Professional Help" frequently. Talk regularly with the person about his or her feelings, just as you do about physical symptoms. Some people find it helpful to rate their anxiety on a 10-point scale, with 0 indicating no anxiety and 10 indicating the worst anxiety ever experienced. Keeping a daily log of anxiety levels takes a little extra effort, but keeping track of anxiety will help you deal with any problems before they get severe.

It usually takes time to deal with anxiety. Look for small improvements at first. Remember that your efforts are successful even if they just stop the anxiety from getting worse. If your efforts do not seem to be helping and the person with cancer has been feeling anxious for several weeks, seek professional help.

CHAPTER EIGHT

Depression

Many people with cancer become depressed at some time during their illness, and family caregivers may become depressed as well. Caregivers often report that dealing with the depression and distressing emotions of the person with cancer was the most difficult symptom they had to deal with during the illness. You can be helpful in controlling symptoms of mild depression. If depression becomes severe, professional help will be needed, and you should encourage the depressed person to get help. In all cases, working together as a team is essential. Paying attention to your own emotional needs is also important and will allow you to give the best possible care.

What Is Depression?

Most people with cancer and their caregivers experience feelings of sadness. Sometimes people are able to get over these feelings after a short time. When these feelings do not go away and last a long time, however, they can severely hurt quality of life. When a person is sad, discouraged, pessimistic, or despairing for several weeks or months and when those feelings interfere with day-to-day activities, that is depression. Depression can last a long time if nothing is done to treat it. There are ways to treat depression, however, and the person can be helped significantly through antidepressant medicines, counseling, and emotional support.

In addition to feelings of sadness, symptoms of depression sometimes include loss of appetite, sleeping problems (either sleeping too much or trouble sleeping), fatigue, and attention or concentration problems. Alcohol abuse may be a sign of depression, especially if it is recent or has worsened since the illness. Sometimes a depressed person thinks about suicide as a way out.

If the person with cancer is depressed, he or she will have problems coping with cancer and the impact it has on his or her life. Depression works like a downward spiral. The person feels down and so does not put energy into solving problems. When problems get worse, the person feels more depressed. Somehow this downward spiral has to be interrupted. A change must happen or the depression will continue for a long time.

Causes of Depression

Depression can be a side effect of some medicines, it can be caused by unrelieved pain, or it can be caused by chemical imbalances in the body due to the cancer. When chemical imbalances happen, a change in treatment may help treat the depression. This chapter covers important warning signs that are present when a depressed person needs medical help. It also covers some strategies to help limit or manage depression. Your help is valuable to a person feeling depressed, but it is also important that he or she practice self-help strategies. This chapter outlines several ways you and the person with cancer can work together as a team to deal with depression.

Feeling down is a normal response to the stresses and uncertainties of chronic illness. Do not expect to get rid of all negative feelings; however, you can help limit the length and severity of depression.

When to Get Professional Help

Get assistance from a health care professional if any of the following conditions exist:

- ***The person talks about hurting or killing himself or herself.*** Suicide is not common among people with cancer—but it is more common among depressed people. Anyone who talks about suicide should be taken seriously. If the person has not made specific remarks but you are concerned, ask if he or she is thinking about suicide. Your asking will not make the person more likely to hurt him or herself. If you believe there is a possibility of suicide, seek professional help immediately. Although it may be uncomfortable for you, it is crucial that you seek professional assistance.
- ***He or she has experienced depression before this illness and has had at least two of the following symptoms consistently during the past two weeks:***
  - feeling sad most of the day
  - loss of interest in almost all daily activities
  - difficulty paying attention to what he or she is doing
  - trouble making choices

People with a history of depression before a serious illness are vulnerable to depression after a major life stress. A serious illness such as cancer can trigger depression. Professional help is usually required.

- ***You notice wide mood swings from periods of depression to periods of agitation and high energy.*** Wide, uncontrollable mood swings can be a symptom of manic-depressive illness. The person may cycle between depressive, low-energy periods and periods of high energy, usually accompanied with feelings of agitation or feeling high or elated. The moods often don't seem connected to what is going on around the person. This condition requires professional help to determine whether medication is necessary.

- **Nothing you do seems to help, even strategies that may have worked in the past.** Health care professionals will be able to help determine the causes of the depression and offer additional treatment recommendations.

Getting help for depression is just like getting help for physical problems. Asking for professional help when needed is not a sign of weakness. The problem could be caused by the stress related to cancer, by the treatment itself, or it could be an understandable reaction to the issues the person is facing.

Some people are hesitant to ask for help with emotional problems because they are embarrassed. They may think seeing a psychologist, psychiatrist, or social worker means they are weak or strange. Being upset during a major illness is normal, as is getting help to deal with these problems.

Ask for help from the doctor who is treating the cancer, a family doctor, or another physician who is familiar with the patient's medical treatments. Physicians familiar with the person's medical condition and treatments can evaluate whether the depression is due to the disease or the treatment. If it is due to the treatment, a change in treatment may be needed. Physicians can also evaluate whether antidepressant medications may help and can prescribe them if necessary. They can also make referrals to mental health professionals.

You can also consult a mental health professional, such as a social worker, psychiatric or mental health nurse, psychologist, or psychiatrist for help. Mental health professionals are experienced in helping people with many types of emotional problems. They can be especially helpful when there is a history of depression before the illness and when the depression is not caused directly by the person's disease or treatments. Many mental health professionals have experience working with people with cancer. They can be very helpful when depression is a reaction to the stress of the illness. Many insurance plans require a referral from the primary care physician. Check whether a referral is required in your situation.

Treating depression takes time. It usually takes several sessions with a counselor or therapist before a person begins to feel better. It also takes time for medicines to work, and the doctor may need to adjust the doses before the medicines for depression are effective.

What You Can Do

You can help manage depression by following these guidelines:

- **Take care of your own emotional needs.**

- **Help the person to recognize and manage mild depression or depressed feelings.**
- **Encourage the person to take part in enjoyable and distracting activities.**
- **Use techniques for controlling negative thoughts.**

Take Care of Your Own Emotional Needs

Living with a person who is depressed can be stressful and can even lead you to become depressed. It is important to pay attention to your own emotional health if you are to do your best as a caregiver. You can also use the ideas in this chapter to monitor your own emotional health and be alert to symptoms of depression.

Depression happens frequently among persons with cancer. However, family members and friends who are caring for someone with cancer often experience depression as well. High levels of stress can make a person feel burned-out. If you feel drained, it is more difficult to help another person. Caregiving can be stressful. To do your best in this difficult role, you need to find ways to stay emotionally well. There are several things you can do for your own emotional health:

Understand that it is not your fault if the person becomes depressed.

You are not responsible for the person's depression. Many things, including biological changes, side effects of treatment, and the stress of illness, can cause depression. Sometimes only professionals can help, especially if the depression is severe. Do not feel guilty if, in spite of your best efforts, the person with cancer becomes or stays depressed.

Schedule positive experiences for yourself.

Keep doing things that make you feel good. Do not become so involved in your caring responsibilities that you neglect your own emotional health. Do not feel guilty about taking care of yourself. If you are overwhelmed, you can't provide adequate care and support. You will be a better caregiver if you take care of yourself and take time to do things you enjoy. Follow this advice early on, and it can help to prevent depressed feelings and give you the strength you need to carry on. Social workers can help you arrange for care so you can take time off. Family or friends may be able to provide care while you take some time for yourself—do not be afraid to ask.

Get the companionship you need.

Remember that you need companionship. Being with others is as important for you as for the person with cancer. Continue to do things with people you like and enjoy. Social interaction helps to prevent and manage your own negative feelings. If you feel yourself becoming depressed, seek out other people for support and companionship. Some people find it helpful to talk to other people about their problems. Look for a support group for caregivers in your community where you can talk about your problems with others who understand your situation. Some people find it more helpful to talk about things that have nothing to do with their problems. That depends on you and what you need.

⫸ You can get professional help for yourself, too, if necessary.

Being a caregiver is a difficult and stressful job, and you may find that you also need the help of a mental health professional to cope with your stress and responsibilities. Do not hesitate to seek out help when you need it.

Help the Person to Recognize and Manage Mild Depression or Depressed Feelings

This section describes several ways to help the person recognize and manage mild depression. Your role as caregiver is twofold: (1) to be a team member by helping the person you are caring for learn these strategies and (2) to be supportive and encouraging about their use. Remember, if depression is severe or ongoing, professional help is needed. The suggestions in this section can help to manage a mild short-term depression, but they cannot prevent or "fix" depression.

⫸ Acknowledge that the person is depressed.

Don't ignore the person's depression. Sometimes people ignore the depression, either because they don't want to encourage it or because they don't want to deal with it. This behavior is not healthy. It may be uncomfortable to acknowledge that someone you love is depressed, but ignoring depression only makes it worse. The depressed person may feel you do not care about his or her feelings.

⫸ Support positive thinking and practice giving helpful responses.

A depressed person might say, "Nothing is going right." Though it may feel that way, there is usually something that is going okay. You can say, "I understand you're feeling discouraged, but let's think of some of the things that are going right." The depressed person might say, "I'm a total failure." The person may feel that way, but you know that his or her whole life is not a failure. You might say, "Maybe you've failed at some things, but think of all the things you have accomplished," and then talk about several of them. Encourage him or her to talk with a health professional who understands the person's condition and treatments.

⫸ Set reasonable, attainable goals.

Depressed people tend to set goals that are too high. Then when they don't reach their goals, they become even more depressed. When you plan positive experiences, be sure that the goals are reasonable. It is better to set a low goal and accomplish more than expected than to set an unrealistic goal and fail. Take as your motto, "Start low and go slow." For example, watch a thirty-minute television show together, listen to a thirty-minute radio show together, ask a friend to drop by for a short visit, or make something easy like pudding and enjoy eating it together.

▦➡ Let the person with cancer know when you think he or she is doing things that may lead to depression.

Making a plan can help the person manage depression early, before it becomes severe. Some people find it helpful to use an agreed upon code word or phrase to point out depressed thinking. However you do it, a gentle reminder to stop and think about negative thoughts can help prevent depression from setting in. In addition, being aware of the person's behavior and negative thoughts can help alert you if professional help is needed.

Encourage the Person to Take Part in Enjoyable and Distracting Activities

Low-level depression (feeling sad or blue) can result from the stress of dealing with cancer. If the person seems to be feeling blue, encourage him or her to do activities that have been pleasant and engaging in the past. Visiting with friends and doing things with other people can be helpful. Tell the person that you care about his or her feelings and that you want to help. Keep in mind that the depressed person is in charge of his or her actions, and your role is to encourage and support.

▦➡ Increase the number of activities involving other people.

Being with people you enjoy is an excellent way to take attention away from negative thoughts and feelings. It provides opportunities to recognize the good aspects of one's life. It also provides opportunities to give and receive help, to share experiences and perspectives, and to get help in dealing with problems. Most important, being surrounded by helpful, loving people can help the person with cancer to face this difficult time with additional strength and confidence.

▦➡ Turn to friends and family members who have helpful qualities.

Think of the people in your lives who are sympathetic and understanding, who give good advice, who can help solve problems, and who can turn attention away from problems and toward pleasant experiences. Think of how to make a visit pleasant and rewarding for them, and then reach out to them and ask for their help. For example, serve a snack or play a game of cards and bring up your difficulties.

▦➡ Encourage the person to substitute positive thoughts and experiences for negative, repetitive thinking.

If the person with cancer is trying to break out of depressive thought patterns, you can help by being encouraging and becoming involved. This support can be as simple as talking about something pleasant or doing an activity together. The next section outlines some techniques for stopping or controlling negative thoughts.

➠ Help the person solve any day-to-day problems that cause stress and may contribute to feelings of depression.
By using a problem-solving approach, you can help the person with cancer deal with household tasks or family matters that are worrying them. For example, the person with cancer may be very stressed about paying bills. Make a plan to do this together and get others to help if needed. Decide who will gather the bills and who will go through them to determine when they are due, and then help the person pay the bills.

➠ Try journaling as an outlet for feelings.
Journaling can help prevent sadness from turning into depression Also known as "personal writing," journaling permits people to write openly about their feelings and concerns. Writing can help you organize your thoughts, gain insight into your feelings, and come up with ideas to better manage situations. The simple suggestions below can help you or the person with cancer get started with journaling:
1. Choose a time and place where you can be comfortable and undisturbed for about fifteen minutes each day.
2. Sit for a couple of minutes and relax before you start writing.
3. Think about the events of the day, and write about anything that comes to your mind. What made you upset or joyful? What are your goals or needs? What have you learned? What are you curious about? What are you grateful for? Don't worry about grammar or punctuation, and try not to criticize or censor your thoughts. A journal is your private space to explore your feelings and thoughts, and there is no right or wrong way to feel. Write as little or as much as you want, and don't worry if you skip a day or two. Writing and then reading your thoughts can help you to gain perspective about your situation and your feelings.

➠ Get help before the depression becomes severe.
If you ignore the early signs of depression, it is more likely to become severe, to seriously affect the quality of life of the person with cancer, and to require professional help.

Use Techniques for Controlling Negative Thoughts

One of the hard things about depression is that it's so easy to get stuck in a whirlwind of negative thinking. Suddenly, you may find depressing thoughts going around and around in your head. It doesn't take long for this pattern to make you feel bad, and then it may seem like you can't stop it. But you can.

If you are feeling depressed, you may look at techniques like these and think they're silly. It may seem impossible that they could work. Research has shown, however, that they can work. Give them a try.

⫸ Use thought-stopping techniques.

Using a thought-stopping technique helps you snap out of it when the whirlwind of negative thoughts starts. If you catch yourself early, you can keep yourself from getting derailed. The trick is to stop negative thoughts when they first begin. When you notice the beginnings of a negative-thinking whirlwind, try one of these techniques:

Yell "STOP!" really loudly in your mind.

When you scream "stop" in your mind, pretend it is very loud. The goal is to wake you up, to make you aware that you are in danger of getting stuck in a negative thought pattern. You might start by going to a place by yourself and shouting "STOP" out loud. Practice it this way until you can do it in your mind alone. It may help to visualize a big red stop sign. Think of what a stop sign looks like, and try to see it clearly. Make sure you see it as a red sign. Practice seeing it in your mind so you can picture it easily. Then whenever you catch yourself starting negative thoughts, think of this image and stop yourself.

Snap your wrist with a rubber band.

Another way to remind yourself to stop negative thoughts is to gently snap your wrist with a rubber band. This technique is not designed to punish negative thinking. Instead, this action can serve as a physical reminder to help you stop the negative thoughts.

Splash some water on your face.

Splashing water in your face is another way to wake yourself up from the negative thinking. Pay attention to how the water makes you feel.

Get up and move to a new spot.

Getting up and moving to a new spot provides a change of scenery. You can use the new surroundings to help you think about more positive things.

Start a pleasant, involving activity.

The activity should take all your attention and push out the negative thinking.

Arrange a time and a place for negative thinking.
This technique allows you to think about and process negative feelings, but it puts you in control of when and where you deal with these thoughts.

Find a negative-thinking "office."
Your "office" space can be any place you choose. It can be a room, a chair, or a certain window. Now try to limit your negative thinking to this one designated place. Do not, however, make it your bed or the place where you eat. Those places need to be safe from negative thinking.

Write down your negative thoughts on a piece of paper.
This step can help you to see your thoughts in perspective. Then rip the paper into small pieces and throw it away.

Schedule a time each day for negative thoughts.
Scheduling a time for negative thoughts helps you to take control of them. You might not be able to control all negative thinking, especially in the beginning, but this technique will gradually help you gain control over your negative thinking. Do not choose a time that is near mealtimes, just before you go to sleep, or just before you expect to see people. Those times should be relaxing. Allow no more than fifteen minutes. At the end of the fifteen minutes, stop. You can continue tomorrow at the same time.

▥▶ Distract yourself.
It is not possible to think about two things at once. When you start to think negatively, get your mind involved in another activity that pushes out or replaces the negative thinking. Try one of these ideas:

- ***Take a vacation in your mind.*** Close your eyes and think about your favorite spot. Spend a couple of minutes there on a mental vacation. Relax and enjoy it.
- ***Mentally travel into the future.*** Think of something you are looking forward to doing. Imagine it is happening. Think of how nice it is to be there.

When you are distracting yourself with time travel or a mental vacation, really try to work your imagination and include as many details as possible. Think about the following questions:

- What does it feel like? Is there a warm breeze? Imagine how it feels on your skin.
- What does it sound like? Are there waves gently crashing on the beach? Are people laughing or is music playing? Imagine it as clearly and vividly as you can.

- What does it look like? Is the sky clear and blue? Are you in a room? Imagine what the room looks like. Try to see it as completely as you can.
- What does it smell like? Is it the salty smell of the ocean? Maybe you smell the fragrances of a garden or a big dinner.
- What does it taste like? Are you drinking a nice cool drink? Feel it in your mouth. Taste it.

Use these exercises to fill your mind with as many pleasant details as you can. This exercise also can be helpful when you are feeling anxious or you are having difficulty falling asleep.

Ⅲ➡ Argue against negative thoughts.

You can fight negative thoughts and challenge their accuracy. Every situation has at least two sides to it. When you are depressed, you may see only the negative, even though things are usually not as bad as they may seem. The only way to see the other side is to actively argue against your own negative thinking. This exercise forces you to take the other side. Think of it as having a debate with yourself.

- ***Begin by asking yourself, "Is my negative thought really true?"***
  Look clearly at the evidence that supports it.
- ***Now take the other side.***
  Argue the exact opposite. Think of every reason why your thought may not be true or may be exaggerated. Don't give up too easily. Really argue as if you were going point-by-point through a debate with someone else.
- ***When you're arguing with your negative thoughts, try to be as complete as possible.***
  You may want to write down the answers to the following questions:
  - What is the evidence against my negative thought?
  - Are there any "facts" in my thinking that are really just assumptions?
  - Is my argument an example of black-and-white thinking? Are there shades of gray that I'm ignoring?
  - Is the negative side taking things out of context? Am I looking at the whole picture or just one small part of it?
  - Am I trying to predict the future when I really know that I can't?
- ***Try to punch as many holes in your "negative sides" argument as you can.***
  Don't accept any illogical thinking.

Possible Challenges

Consider the following situations that have been difficult for other caregivers:

"I don't want your help. Leave me alone."

Let the person know that you need their cooperation and participation in order for the plan to be effective. Assure him or her that you will not do anything without his or her agreement and cooperation. Starting small with something that is easy to do may seem more amenable to the person. If the person is unwilling to try anything, you should seek professional help.

"My problems are real! It's normal to be depressed in my situation."

Agree that the person's problems are real and some sadness is normal. However, getting stuck in the feeling of depression can interfere with dealing with the problems that are causing the depression. The goal is to keep a balance between positive and negative thoughts. The problems are real, but many of the good things in life are also real and should get equal attention.

"Nothing will help, so it's no use trying."

While it may seem that way to the person, assure him or her that those types of thoughts are the depression talking. Encourage him or her to try. There is nothing to lose and a good deal to gain. You can start with small, manageable things that are easy to do and then decide whether these ideas are helpful. If the person is unwilling to try, seek professional help.

Carrying Out and Adjusting Your Plan

Think of other challenges that could interfere with your plans to manage depression. What additional roadblocks could get in the way of following the recommendations in this chapter? Will the person with cancer talk about his or her feelings? Will other people listen? How will you explain your needs to medical professionals? Do you have the time and energy to carry out the plan? Develop plans for getting around these roadblocks using the COPE ideas discussed in the introduction.

Talk with the person about the ideas in this chapter. Agree on what you can do together to manage depression. It is important to work as a team when dealing with these problems. Sometimes support and the feeling of being on a team is in itself helpful to a depressed person.

- **Use these techniques early.** Watch for the beginning signs of depression, and put your plan into action immediately. Don't wait until depression is severe. The techniques discussed in this chapter have helped severely depressed people, but usually as part of professional treatment. As a caregiver, you can help the person with cancer the most by acting before depression becomes severe.

- ***Plan in advance what you will do to manage depression.*** If you know the person with cancer is likely to be depressed at certain times based on past experience, make plans for what you will do to prevent depression from worsening.
- ***Persist.*** Even if the person continues to feel depressed, don't give up. Try other techniques recommended in this chapter and seek professional help if the condition worsens.

Talk regularly with the person with cancer about his or her feelings. Although it may be difficult for you at first, let the person with cancer know you understand depression can happen during illness. If you show you are comfortable talking about feelings, the person with cancer is more likely to let you know if he or she is experiencing depressive symptoms. It may seem scary at first to talk about problems, but it is important to listen. It shows you care, and it also helps you work together as a team to manage negative thoughts and feelings. Watch for indications that professional help is needed.

Ask yourself if you are expecting change too fast. It can take time for depression to improve. Look for small improvements. Remember that your efforts can be successful even if they just keep the depression from getting worse.

If the coping strategies in this chapter are not helping and the person has been feeling very depressed for several weeks, encourage the person to seek professional help.

Part III

Physical Side Effects of Cancer and Cancer Treatment

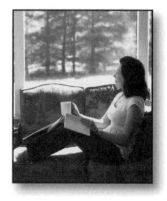

THIS SECTION ADDRESSES SOME OF THE COMMON SIDE EFFECTS OF CANCER AND/OR CANCER TREATMENT. Chapter topics include nausea and vomiting, constipation, diarrhea, fever and infections, pain, mouth problems, skin problems, loss of appetite, bleeding, tiredness and fatigue, sleep problems, and hair loss. Understanding these conditions and being prepared to deal with them will help you and the person with cancer work together to solve problems.

This section also addresses some less common conditions or situations that can occur while the person is undergoing cancer treatment: mobility problems and falls, problems with veins and vein punctures, and confusion and seizures. Mobility issues may come up during treatment, and it is very important for a caregiver to understand how best to create a safe environment and know what to do if the person falls. Some people with cancer will have problems—physical or psychological—with vein punctures because of frequent blood tests and/or the use of veins for chemotherapy. And finally, confusion and seizures are not common, but they may occur.

Each person's experience with cancer and cancer treatment is unique, and no one can predict how they will affect your loved one. Not everyone experiences side effects with treatment, and, for those who do, not everyone has the same side effects or reacts to treatment in the same way.

This section is primarily organized to help you deal with problems or side effects that may come up during cancer treatment and caregiving. Each chapter is organized under five major topics:

1. Understanding the condition
   - when the problem will likely occur
   - what kinds of things can be done to help
   - what goals to have when dealing with the condition

2. When to get professional help
   - when to call for help immediately
   - when to call during office hours
   - what information to have ready when you're calling

3. What you can do
   - what you can do to manage the problem at home
   - what you can do to help to prevent the problem

4. Possible challenges
   - recognizing problems
   - how to deal with problems you may have in carrying out your plans

5. Carrying out and adjusting the plan
   - how to monitor progress
   - how quickly to expect change
   - what to do if the plan isn't working

The information in this section fits most situations, but your situation may be different. If the person's doctor or nurse provides different instructions, always follow the advice of your health care providers. For more information on coping with cancer and cancer treatment, contact the American Cancer Society at **800-227-2345** or visit the Web site at **cancer.org**.

CHAPTER NINE

Nausea and Vomiting

It's natural for someone preparing for cancer treatment to be concerned about nausea and vomiting. They are very uncomfortable symptoms many people associate with cancer treatment. A great deal has been learned, however, about how to control both nausea and vomiting. Most people receiving treatments for cancer today have much less nausea and vomiting than patients in the past.

Some people do not experience any nausea or vomiting as a result of cancer or its treatments. Other people deal with one or both symptoms at different times in their illness, depending on which treatments they receive and their reactions to them. Sometimes, if treatment has caused nausea, the person may feel nauseated when he or she sees or smells something associated with the treatment. For example, the smell of the treatment room or the sight of the nurse or doctor who administered the treatments may cause nausea or even vomiting. This reaction is normal and will usually go away after treatments are over. It is a learned association between the sights and smells of treatment and feeling nauseated.

When to Get Professional Help

Ask the doctor or nurse to help you fill in the blanks below, and call them if any of the following conditions exist:

- ***There is blood or material that looks like coffee grounds in the vomit.*** Material that looks like coffee grounds is actually old blood and signals that there has been bleeding inside the body. This is rare, but it is important to report if it happens.
- ***Vomiting occurs more than _____ times an hour for more than _____ hours.*** Ask the doctor or nurse to fill in the blanks with the appropriate times. For most people, vomiting three times per hour for more than twelve hours is serious, but it may be different for the person for whom you are caring.
- ***The vomit shoots out a distance or with great force (projectile vomiting).*** Projectile

vomiting may mean there are problems in the stomach or intestine that should be investigated by the doctor.

- **The person has missed or vomited up to two doses of any prescribed medicines.** Medicines will have to be given other ways until pills can stay down again.
- **Fewer than ___ cups of liquid are consumed in twenty-four hours and no solid food is eaten.** Ask the doctor or nurse to help you fill in the blank space above. Vomiting can cause dehydration, especially if the person is unable to drink or keep down liquids. Food is also needed to keep up the person's energy and to fight illness. Most people need to drink more than four cups of liquid in twenty-four hours. Also, for most people, two days without food is dangerous. The needs of the person for whom you are caring may be different, however, so ask the doctor or nurse when to call about this problem.
- **Weakness or dizziness occurs with the nausea or vomiting.** It is normal to feel a little weak or dizzy with nausea, but if the person can't get up, you need to call the doctor or nurse.
- **Severe stomach pain occurs with vomiting.** Severe pain is always a reason to call the doctor immediately.

Have the following information available before you call the doctor or nurse:
- How long has nausea been a problem?
- When did it begin and how long has it lasted?
- How bad was the most recent nausea?
- How much does the nausea interfere with normal activities?
- Was medicine prescribed for nausea or vomiting?
  - Name of medicine(s)
  - How often should it be taken?
  - How many pills at one time?
  - How many pills were taken in the last two days?
  - How much relief did it give?
  - How long did the relief last?
- Were any nonprescription medicines taken for the nausea? If so, what were they and what were the results?
- In addition to giving medicine for nausea, what was done to help the person with nausea feel better and what were the results?
- Was the nausea followed by vomiting?
- What did the vomit look like? Was this vomit the same color as earlier vomit? If not, how was it different?
- How often has vomiting happened in the last twenty-four hours?

- What other symptoms are new since the nausea or vomiting began? (Answer questions below for each new symptom.)
  - Where in the body is it?
  - How bad is it?
  - When did it start?
  - When does it happen?
  - How long does it last?
  - What relieves it?
  - What doesn't help?
- What and how much was eaten in the last twenty-four hours?
- What and how much liquid was consumed in the last twenty-four hours?
- How frequent were bowel movements in the last two days, and were they the same amount and color as usual? Has the person taken laxatives or stool softeners recently?
- What is the persons' temperature?
- When was the last cancer treatment, and was there anything new or different about the last treatment?

What You Can Do

You can manage nausea and vomiting by following these guidelines:

- **Make the best use of anti-nausea medicines.**
- **Do what you can to ease nausea and vomiting.**

Make the Best Use of Anti-nausea Medicines

As with any medication, be sure you follow the instructions on the label and the instructions given by the nursing staff. Encourage the person experiencing nausea to follow these guidelines:

Take anti-nausea medicine on a regular schedule.

Most anti-nausea medicine must be taken on a regular schedule (not just when nausea occurs) to maintain enough of the medicine in the blood to be effective.

Take anti-nausea medicines half an hour before meals.

Anti-nausea medicine often helps with appetite in people suffering from nausea.

Take anti-nausea medicine before and after receiving chemotherapy treatments.

Anti-nausea medicine should be taken before chemotherapy and then continued every four to six hours or as directed by the doctor. A sample dosage schedule might look like this:

- Take at bedtime the night before treatment.
- Take in the morning before treatment.
- Take four to six hours after treatment for at least twelve to twenty-four hours. Continue on that schedule as long as nausea or vomiting persists. You can use table 9.1 to chart the times at which medicine should be taken.

Table 9.1. Anti-nausea Medication Schedule														
DAY		**HOUR**												
		12	1	2	3	4	5	6	7	8	9	10	11
MONDAY	A.M.												
	P.M.												
TUESDAY	A.M.												
	P.M.												
WEDNESDAY	A.M.												
	P.M.												
THURSDAY	A.M.												
	P.M.												
FRIDAY	A.M.												
	P.M.												
SATURDAY	A.M.												
	P.M.												
SUNDAY	A.M.												
	P.M.												

Do What You Can to Ease Nausea and Vomiting

Consider the following ideas to help reduce nausea and vomiting. Start with ideas that have helped in the past, but try new ideas, too. You can't know whether something will help until you try it. Encourage the person with cancer to do the following:

➤ Eat three to four hours before treatment but not just before treatment.

Eating frequent light meals during the day keeps something in the stomach and helps the body get the nutrition it needs. For some people, having the stomach empty just before treatments can help reduce nausea.

➤ Don't eat fried foods, dairy products, and acids such as fruit juices or salad dressings with vinegar.

If you are experiencing nausea, avoid these foods. Fried and acidic foods are hard to digest and may make nausea worse.

➤ Try chewing gum, hard candy, or candied ginger.

Try hard mints or fruit-flavored candies or gums. They cover up unpleasant tastes during chemotherapy. Candied ginger can also help reduce nausea but shouldn't be eaten in large quantities.

➤ Let fresh air into the house or go outside.

Taking in more oxygen can decrease feelings of nausea. Open a window or door to let fresh air into the house. Encourage the person to breathe through the mouth for a few minutes.

➤ Rest.

Some people find it helpful to lie down when they are nauseated. Anti-nausea medicine often makes people sleepy, which helps them rest through their nausea. Allow short rest times between everyday activities such as dressing or walking. Taking it easy can help reduce feelings of nausea.

➤ Sip fluids two hours after vomiting.

Wait a while after the person has vomited before offering food or drink. Then offer one or two ounces of fluid at a time. Let the fizz go out of sodas before drinking them—carbonation can upset the stomach. Stir sodas vigorously with a spoon to release carbonation, or leave the can open or the cap off for a time.

➤ Eat dry crackers.

Bland foods are easy to digest and may help stave off nausea. Nauseated people may find eating a few dry crackers calms the stomach.

▐▶ **Avoid unpleasant or strong odors.**

It may help the person with cancer to stay away from the kitchen. Suggest breathing through the mouth and not through the nose to minimize strong odors.

▐▶ **Rinse the mouth frequently.**

Frequent swishing and rinsing remove unpleasant tastes that can upset the stomach.

▐▶ **Wear loosely fitting clothes.**

Avoid tight-fitting clothing, especially around the waist or neck. Tight-fitting garments put pressure on the throat and stomach and can add to stomach upset.

▐▶ **Try distracting activities.**

Watching television, listening to music, or reading may help distract the person with nausea.

▐▶ **Relax.**

If the person with cancer is tense, physical symptoms also can seem more intense. Many people find that relaxing helps to ease symptoms. (Refer to the chapter on anxiety for a detailed explanation of how to practice relaxation techniques.)

▐▶ **Go to treatments with another person.**

A companion can show support and help the person with cancer think and talk about things besides nausea and treatment. A companion can also encourage relaxation exercises and even be a coach during exercises.

Possible Challenges

Consider the following situation that has been difficult for another caregiver:

"My husband takes medicines for other health problems that make him sick to his stomach, and he can't stop taking those other pills. What can I do about that?"

If the person with cancer must take other medication, never give them on an empty stomach unless the label instructs you to do so. Otherwise, offer a medicine such as Maalox, dry bread, or saltine crackers beforehand, or give the medicine after a meal. If the person with nausea is taking potassium pills or potassium liquid, talk with the pharmacist or nurse about its side effects. Potassium can cause nausea, which can make the nausea from chemotherapy worse. Ask the doctor about different ways to take potassium that may not cause as much nausea.

Carrying Out and Adjusting Your Plan

Think of other challenges that could interfere with carrying out your plan to manage nausea and vomiting. What additional roadblocks could get in the way of following the recommendations in this chapter? Will the person with cancer take anti-nausea medicines? Will other people accompany the person with cancer to treatments? How will you explain your needs to medical professionals? Do you have the time and energy to carry out the plan? Develop plans for getting around these challenges by using the COPE ideas discussed in the introduction.

Keep track of how the person is doing by monitoring how often the person vomits, the severity of his or her nausea, and how much he or she cuts back on normal activities because of nausea. You can create a table such as the example in table 9.2 to help keep track.

Table 9.2. Rating Vomiting and Nausea			
DAY	**VOMITING**[a]	**NAUSEA**[b]	**INTERFERENCE WITH ACTIVITIES**[c]
MONDAY			
TUESDAY			
WEDNESDAY			
THURSDAY			
FRIDAY			
SATURDAY			
SUNDAY			

[a] Record number of times person vomited.

[b] Rate severity of nausea: 0 = not at all severe; 5 = moderately severe; 10 = very severe.

[c] Rate amount of interference with activities: 0 = did not require cutting back activities at all; 5 = required cutting back activities moderately; 10 = required cutting back all activities.

If nausea and vomiting are getting worse, review the section "When to Get Professional Help" on page 95. Ask yourself if you are doing everything you can to reduce this symptom. If the person is becoming anxious about nausea or the nausea is becoming harder to control, ask the doctor about other anti-nausea medicines, reducing the chemotherapy dose, or other methods to cope with nausea and vomiting.

CHAPTER TEN

Constipation

Most constipation can be prevented, but prevention takes planning and attention to the person's diet. It may also involve taking preventive medicine if it is prescribed. As the caregiver, you are key to managing and preventing this uncomfortable condition. Because constipation is a sensitive subject for many people, tact and sensitivity are important when providing care. You will need to communicate clearly and sensitively with the person and keep in close contact with health care professionals to manage this problem.

Constipation occurs when bowel movements happen less often than usual and when stools are hard or difficult to move. Constipation can be caused by medicines used to treat cancer, opioids used to ease pain, emotional stress, changes in diet, or decreases in activity. Constipation is a common problem for people who are weak, are spending a lot of time in bed, or are not eating very much. Even if the person with cancer isn't eating much, however, the body still makes waste, and regular bowel movements are necessary.

Constipation can be very uncomfortable. A constipated person may have a decreased appetite, feel bloated, or have abdominal cramps. These feelings add to the person's overall discomfort.

When to Get Professional Help

It is important to report constipation to the doctor or nurse because this symptom could indicate other problems. For example, a tumor could be pressing on a part of the bowel and preventing stool from passing through it normally.

Call the doctor or nurse if any of the following conditions exist:
- ***The normal bowel routine is disrupted.*** Perhaps the routine was once a day, and he or she has not had a bowel movement in three or four days. Or perhaps the normal rou-

tine was once every other day, and he or she has not had a bowel movement in four or five days. Constipation becomes more uncomfortable as it continues. If it continues for more than a few days, it will also be more difficult to reverse.

- ***The person is experiencing severe straining on the toilet.***
- ***The patient experiences severe abdominal pain, the abdomen feels harder than normal, or there is blood in the stool.*** These signs can mean that the constipation needs medical attention.

When you call the health care provider, it is important to give as much detail as possible. Report all the symptoms, the person's usual bowel pattern, and the day and type of the last movement. This information helps the doctor or nurse decide what medicines could help and advise you on other measures to help relieve the problem. For example, signs such as smears of stool on the person's underwear or a feeling of fullness in the rectal area can indicate to the doctor that the lower bowel needs to be evacuated. In that case, the doctor would likely prescribe a laxative or stool softener to help with emptying the lower bowel in the future.

The doctor or nurse may ask you the following questions, which help them assess whether constipation is getting worse and whether there is stool close to the rectum that is not being moved by the necessary muscles.

Have the following information available when you call the doctor or nurse:
- How often does the person usually have bowel movements?
- When was the last bowel movement? What did it look like? Reporting what the last bowel movement looked like (watery or dry) tells the health professional whether food is being digested properly and whether the stool has enough water in it as it passes through the digestive tract. Color also is important to report. Very dark stools could indicate blood in the stool.
- Does the person normally take medicines to help move the bowels, such as laxatives, stool softeners, fiber supplements, herbal mixtures, or suppositories? If yes, what kind and how often are they used?
- Do feelings of constipation interfere with normal activities, such as walking or eating? The degree to which the constipation interferes with the person's comfort and activities is important to report because this information indicates how severe the constipation is and how important it is to treat quickly.
- What other symptoms are there?
  - distention or bloating of the abdomen
  - pressure or sense of fullness in the rectal area
  - small, frequent smears of stool on the person's underwear

- small amounts of loose stools, diarrhea, or leaking
- rectal pain with a bowel movement
- constantly feeling the need to have a bowel movement but unable to pass stool
- nausea
- blood in the stools or dark or black stools

Answers to questions about other symptoms help the doctors and nurses understand the condition. If there is no bowel movement for days, but small amounts of diarrhea occur, they may recommend a gentle enema or a visit to the clinic for a rectal exam and further assessment.

- What medications were taken in the last two to three days? Be sure to mention any medicines the person is taking, especially narcotics (opioids or pain pills), laxatives, or chemotherapy. Some medicines can interrupt normal bowel activity, and the doctor or nurse will recognize which medicines could be contributing to constipation.
- How much food and liquid was consumed during the last twenty-four hours? If the doctor knows about food and fluid intake, he or she can judge whether the constipation requires a visit to the clinic. If the doctor decides the constipation is not an emergency, he or she may suggest an increase in fluids and some of the actions that are listed on the following pages.

What You Can Do

You can manage constipation by following these guidelines:
- **Relieve constipation.**
- **Prevent constipation.**

Relieve Constipation

A number of things can be done to relieve constipation. Talk to the doctor, however, before taking these steps to determine the most appropriate course of action for the person.

➡ **Talk to the doctor about using stool softeners or oral laxatives that have stool softeners in them every day.**

Talk with the doctor or nurse to determine the best regimen of laxatives or stool softeners. The doctor may recommend starting with two at night and adding additional medicine in the morning if there is no relief. Laxatives relieve constipation by stimulating the bowels to move waste products out of the body. Stool softeners draw water into the bowel and decrease the dryness of stools so that stool moves through the long intestine more easily. The combination of laxatives and stool softeners gives the best results. These medicines can be bought at any pharmacy. There are many brands to choose from, but Senokot tablets are frequently used when constipation is caused by pain medicines. If finances are a concern, ask the pharmacist about less expensive medicines, or ask the doctor or nurse whether you can have office samples.

▸ **If necessary, increase the number of laxative tablets.**

Different people require different amounts of these medicines. If the previous laxative schedule isn't working, ask the doctor or nurse if you can increase the number of tablets. People taking opioid pain medicines may need as many as six to eight pills per day to prevent constipation from the medication. Make sure to read the product label for possible side effects and immediately report any problems to a doctor or nurse. Examples of possible side effects include severe stomach cramping, nausea, or vomiting.

▸ **Use a rectal suppository after checking with the doctor or nurse.**

Suppositories can be inserted in the rectum, where they stimulate the lower bowel to move. Suppositories should be stored in the refrigerator, because they will become soft at room temperature. Suppositories should not be used, however, if the person with cancer has low platelet or white blood cell counts since there is a risk of infection or bleeding if the suppository breaks a blood vessel in the rectal area.

▸ **Use enemas only after checking with the doctor or nurse.**

Give a mineral oil enema, Fleet enema, or soapsuds enema for immediate relief, but first check with the doctor or nurse. Enemas are the last step to relieve constipation. They evacuate the lower bowel, which helps the upper bowel move as well.

- A mineral oil enema softens stool. Usually, a small amount of mineral oil (four ounces) is pushed gently into the bowel through a small plastic bottle. The person then holds the oil in until he or she feels the urge to have a bowel movement.

- A Fleet enema puts about four ounces of chemically treated (sodium phosphate or sodium biphosphate) water into the bowel, along with medicines such as castor oil or laxatives. Fleet enemas are available at most pharmacies.

- A soapsuds enema can be made at home. Mix four to eight ounces of warm water with a small amount of dish soap, and then place this soapy water in a plastic enema bag. Lubricate the end of the bag with oil or Vaseline and insert into the rectum. The soapsuds mixture drips slowly into the lower bowel. The bowels move because the volume of liquid stimulates movement and because the soapsuds mildly irritate the bowel.

All of these enemas and equipment can be bought at a pharmacy. You may be able to buy a small, two-inch enema that is easy to insert and works well. Only one or two enemas are usually needed to relieve constipation. It is best to give an enema with the person lying on his or her left side near a bathroom or with a commode next to the bed or couch.

Prevent Constipation

There are many things you can do to prevent constipation. If the person with cancer has been constipated recently, encourage the use of these strategies to help prevent it in the future:

➠ **Gradually add foods high in fiber to the diet:**
- whole grain cereals and breads
- dried fruits, including prunes and raisins
- popcorn, nuts, and seeds
- beans and legumes
- raw fruits and vegetables

High-fiber foods draw water into the stools. They also provide bulk—that is, they are made of materials that do not break down as the food passes through the intestines, where it is normally dissolved by acids and enzymes. For example, the skins and coverings of nuts, beans, grains, fruits, and vegetables are not easily broken down, and these help form stools that are easily passed out of the body. If raw fruits and vegetables are hard to chew, try grating or cooking them.

➠ **Add unprocessed bran to the diet.**
Bran stimulates bowel activity. Sprinkle it on cereal, or mix it with yogurt, applesauce, or pudding. Start with two teaspoons per day, and gradually work up to two tablespoons per day. Use caution and make sure to increase the amount gradually. Adding large amounts of bran to the diet too quickly can cause gas, diarrhea, and discomfort.

➠ **Drink plenty of fluids, up to six to eight glasses of liquid every day.**
Fluids add water to the stools and prevent constipation caused by dry, hard stools.

➠ **Drink hot or warm liquids.**
Hot or warm liquids stimulate the bowels. People often say that coffee makes them go to the bathroom. The combination of caffeine and hot liquid causes this effect.

➠ **Drink prune juice, hot lemon water, or hot tea.**
Warm or cold prune juice, hot lemon water, and hot tea all stimulate the bowels.

▥➡ **Encourage exercise, such as walking every day.**

Even a small amount of movement, such as walking in the house, helps stimulate the muscles that make the bowel work. Talk to the doctor about the amount and type of exercise that is appropriate for the person with cancer.

▥➡ **Avoid regular use of enemas, if possible.**

Frequent enemas may prevent the intestines from forming a regular bowel pattern.

▥➡ **Talk to the doctor about daily use of stool softeners and/or laxatives—especially if the person is taking opioids.**

If the person is eating or drinking less and not feeling well enough to exercise, talk to the doctor about adding stool softeners to the daily routine. If the person is taking opioids, talk to the doctor about a daily laxative and read the chapter on pain (beginning on page 125) for a more complete explanation of using laxatives with opioids.

Possible Challenges

Consider the following situations that have been difficult for other caregivers:

"She hasn't eaten much all month. How could anything be in there to plug her up or make her constipated?"

The body makes waste products and stool even when people eat very little. Taking narcotics (opioids), not walking much, and not drinking enough fluids make constipation more likely to happen. Laxatives or enemas may be needed to get the bowels moving.

"He's too embarrassed about his constipation to talk to me about it, so how can I help him?"

Put him in charge of his own care. Have him read this chapter. If possible, help him to understand what causes constipation and what to do about it. Then he can be responsible for managing it. Another strategy is to have him talk directly to a nurse. Most people are willing to talk about things that embarrass them to health care professionals. Health care professionals are experienced in discussing these subjects without embarrassment.

Carrying Out and Adjusting Your Plan

Think of other challenges that could interfere with carrying out your plan to manage constipation. What additional roadblocks could get in the way of following the recommendations in this chapter? Will the person with cancer talk about this problem? How will you explain your needs to medical professionals? Do you have the time and energy to carry out the plan? Develop plans for getting around these challenges by using the COPE ideas discussed in the introduction.

Prepare in advance for constipation, especially if opioids are prescribed or if the person is not able to be very active. Make changes to the person's diet and food habits to prevent constipation. After the person starts new medicines, ask if bowel habits are changing or if constipation is getting better or worse. When does constipation happen? Do you both know what to do to relieve it? Are actions to prevent constipation taking effect?

If your plan does not seem to be working or constipation is getting worse, speak with the doctor or nurse. Discuss the results of your plan and ask what additional steps should be taken to manage the problem.

CHAPTER ELEVEN

Diarrhea

Diarrhea is defined as liquid stools. With diarrhea, bowel movements can happen more frequently than usual and feel more urgent. Having diarrhea can be very upsetting. It can be caused by cancer treatments, some other types of medicines, and sometimes emotional distress. Losing fluids through diarrhea adds to fatigue and feeling washed out. Diarrhea also can cause dehydration, which can be serious. Another possible side effect of diarrhea is a rectal infection. Rectal infections can be caused by bacteria that invade the body when the skin is broken from the acids and irritants in the diarrheal stool. This condition is uncomfortable and painful. Therefore, stopping diarrhea is important for both comfort and health.

Diarrhea can have serious health effects, so correct management is important. Be especially alert for dehydration. Get professional help early for severe diarrhea, and encourage the person to drink more fluids. If the person is unable to take care of him- or herself, the caregiver will have to deal with the diarrhea directly, which can be very stressful. If diarrhea continues for a long time, ask others to help you.

When to Get Professional Help

The most critical problem to watch for is **severe diarrhea**. Severe diarrhea means a lot of fluid is being lost. With severe diarrhea, stools are very runny, and the person often complains of stomach cramps as well. The severity of the problem depends on many factors, such as the person's weight or previous state of fluid balance. Losing small amounts of fluid and stool in diarrhea can be dangerous for a small, thin person or for anyone who has recently been struggling with diarrhea or vomiting. In this situation, dehydration happens quickly. Severe diarrhea demands quick attention. Reporting severe diarrhea early is important so medicines and fluids can be given to stop the diarrhea and to reverse or correct dehydration. Serious health problems can result if a person loses too much fluid and gets dehydrated.

In addition, call the doctor or nurse if any of the following conditions exist:

- **Diarrhea for more than one day**
- **Blood in the diarrhea**
- **Fever of 100.5°F or above with diarrhea**

Have the following information available when you call the doctor or nurse:

- How many bowel movements does the person usually have each day?
- How many bowel movements have there been in the last twenty-four hours?
- How runny were they?
- Are there any other symptoms with the diarrhea?
  - stomach pain or cramping
  - bloating (feeling very full in the stomach or abdomen)
  - nausea or vomiting
  - fever
  - blood in the stool
  - other
- In the previous two days, how much liquid and solid food was consumed? Knowing how much food and liquid the person has had helps the doctor and nurse determine whether the body is receiving enough to replace what is being lost. Dehydration can lead to dangerously low blood pressure and chemical imbalances in the body. Sometimes intravenous (IV) fluids are ordered to balance the fluid loss and put important fluids, water, vitamins, and minerals back into the body.
- What medicines were taken in the last two to three days? At what dosage?
  - chemotherapy (when?)
  - laxatives
  - anti-diarrhea tablets or liquids
  - other medicines, including nonprescription and herbal medicines
- Has weight been lost? How much?
- Is there any history of other bowel problems, such as diverticulitis, colitis, or irritable bowel syndrome?

What You Can Do

You can manage diarrhea by following these guidelines:

- **Use medicines for diarrhea.**
- **Replace lost fluids and nutrients after diarrhea.**

- **Discourage eating foods that make diarrhea worse.**
- **Increase comfort.**

Use Medicines for Diarrhea

Using anti-diarrhea medicine is a fast way to stop diarrhea. These medicines slow down the bowel. Encourage the person with cancer to follow these guidelines:

➠ **Check with the doctor or nurse before using over-the-counter anti-diarrhea medicines.**
The doctor might prefer that you use a prescription medicine or certain over-the-counter medicines to stop diarrhea.

➠ **Follow the instructions on the bottle or on the prescription label.**
Sometimes anti-diarrhea medicines do the job too well. If the person takes too much, cramping and constipation can result. The person may get very sleepy if given too much anti-diarrhea medicine.

Replace Lost Fluids and Nutrients After Diarrhea

Important fluids are lost with diarrheal stool, and replacing these fluids is crucial. Try to increase fluid intake to three quarts a day—unless the doctor or nurse says otherwise.

➠ **Drink clear liquids.**
Examples include chicken broth; weak, tepid tea; apple, cranberry, or grape juice; peach nectar; ginger ale; Jell-O; Popsicles; and Gatorade. These drinks and foods provide important nutrients but also let the bowel rest. Clear liquids are easier for the intestines to absorb into the bloodstream, and they help replace the fluids lost with diarrhea.

➠ **Drink fluids between meals.**
Drinking fluids between meals keeps a steady amount of water and other nutrients entering the body.

➠ **Increase high-potassium foods in the diet.**
Try apricot or peach nectar, bananas, and mashed or baked potatoes. People tend to lose potassium when they have diarrhea. This chemical is vital to the body and needs to be replaced.

▥▶ Eat small meals throughout the day instead of three large meals.

Try six small meals in a day. Smaller meals are easier to digest, and the person will often take in more food or liquid with frequent small meals than with three large meals.

Discourage Eating Foods that Make Diarrhea Worse

Some foods increase the action of the bowel and how quickly it pulls fluid out of body tissues into stool. Examples of foods to avoid are greasy and fatty foods, ice cream and milk, beans, and broccoli. Avoiding these foods can help reduce problems with diarrhea.

▥▶ Eat low-fiber foods.

For example, try bananas, rice, applesauce, mashed potatoes, dry toast, crackers, eggs, fish, poultry, cottage cheese, and yogurt (unless dairy foods are problematic). Low-fiber foods do not attract or pull water out of the body into the bowel. They are easier to digest than high-fiber vegetables.

▥▶ Avoid foods that produce gas.

These foods include beans, raw vegetables, raw fruits, broccoli, corn, cabbage, cauliflower, and carbonated drinks. These foods cause a feeling of fullness and can make a person stop eating or drinking earlier. Gas also adds to discomfort. Avoid chewing gum because it makes some people swallow air, which adds to abdominal discomfort.

▥▶ Avoid foods that contain acids.

These foods include citrus juices like orange and grapefruit juice. These acids make the stomach and intestines churn and can cause discomfort and diarrhea.

▥▶ Avoid fats, such as fatty meats and greasy fried foods.

Fats are difficult to digest. If the person has diarrhea, fats will be pushed through the intestines without being digested. Undigested fat increases the amount and frequency of diarrhea.

▥▶ Cool down hot food or hot drinks.

Hot foods and liquids make the bowels move. Avoid hot temperatures until diarrhea ends.

▥▶ Limit caffeine intake.

That means limiting coffee, strong teas, sodas with caffeine, and chocolate. Caffeine makes the bowels work faster. If a person has diarrhea, you want to slow the bowels down.

▐▶ **Avoid milk and milk products if they seem to make diarrhea worse.**
Milk can make diarrhea worse. It can also cause stomach cramps in some adults.

Increase Comfort

The intestinal cramps that may accompany diarrhea can cause the lower abdomen to become sore. The person may also feel worn out from bouts with diarrhea. Rectal skin or the skin around a stoma (an opening in the abdomen from which stool comes out into a bag) can become very sore. There are several ways to ease abdominal or skin soreness. Encourage the person with diarrhea to do the following:

▐▶ **Put a warm water bottle wrapped in a towel on the abdomen.**
Warmth on the stomach can relieve pain and discomfort caused by stomach tightness or cramps. Do not, however, use a heating pad or put very hot water in the water bottle. The skin may be sensitive to heat, especially if the person is undergoing chemotherapy or radiation therapy, and a heating pad or very hot water bottle could cause skin problems.

▐▶ **Cleanse the rectal area after episodes of diarrhea.**
After diarrhea, cleanse the outside of the rectum gently with warm water and then allow the skin to dry to reduce irritation and prevent infection. Always clean the rectal area from front to back so that stool will not be spread toward the opening to the bladder or vagina.

▐▶ **Soak in warm water.**
Use a tub or sitz bath. Sitz baths can be bought at most pharmacies or medical equipment stores. Sitz baths are plastic bowls that fit over the toilet. The person sits in the bowl of warm water, with overflow spilling into the toilet below. Sitting in warm water in the bathtub can also be helpful.

▐▶ **Apply soothing creams, ointments, or astringent pads, such as Tucks, to the rectal area.**
Astringent pads help clean and dry the area and soothe irritated skin. Creams prevent rectal skin from chapping in the same way they prevent diaper rash or chapping on infants' skin. Try brands such as Nupercainal, A&D, or Vaseline.

▐▶ **If diarrhea continues and the rectal area becomes very sore and red, apply an ointment for protection.**
Desitin ointment, for example, protects the skin from irritants in diarrhea. Fluids will be less likely to burn the skin since this type of ointment covers the skin with a protective layer.

▸ **Protect the bed and chairs from being soiled.**

Put two overlapping waterproof pads or Chux (blue disposable underpads) under the buttocks where the person will lie or sit. For the bed, a plastic trash bag under the waterproof pads will give extra protection, as will a plastic mattress pad.

▸ **Talk to an enterostomal therapist (a specially trained nurse) for recommendations if the person with cancer has a stoma and the skin around the opening becomes irritated.**

An enterostomal therapist may have further ideas or suggestions to ease the person's discomfort. This person can also suggest ways to keep the anus and rectum healthy.

Possible Challenges

Consider the following situation that has been difficult for another caregiver:

"He's had nothing to eat or drink for days, so this diarrhea can't last much longer."

The body can continue to remove fluid for much longer than you might think. Fluid is drawn from body tissues, and so diarrhea can continue even if the person stops eating or drinking for days. It's important to replace the fluids that are lost, even if it seems these fluids will be washed out instantly.

Carrying Out and Adjusting Your Plan

Think of other challenges that could interfere with carrying out your plan to manage diarrhea. What additional roadblocks could get in the way of following the recommendations in this chapter? Will the person with cancer cooperate in replenishing lost fluids? Will other people help provide care? How will you explain your needs to medical professionals? Do you have the time and energy to carry out the plan? Develop plans for getting around these challenges by using the COPE ideas discussed in the introduction.

Keep track of the frequency and severity of diarrhea. Are you able to stop the diarrhea when it starts? Is the rectal skin or skin around a stoma well cared for and protected? Are other precautions with fluids and diet being followed to prevent diarrhea? If problems with diarrhea are getting worse or the person with cancer is becoming worn out, review the section "When to Get Professional Help." If diarrhea isn't severe but continues for several days, ask for help. Call the doctor or nurse to discuss the results of your plan and what additional steps should be taken to manage the problem.

CHAPTER TWELVE

Fever and Infections

There are a few things to keep in mind about fevers during cancer treatment. Fevers are a key sign that there is a problem, such as an infection. But fevers can also be a side effect of some medicines or treatments. Fevers can get out of hand quickly, so it is important to be on the look-out for fevers and to act quickly to keep them under control. Fevers can be tiring, and the chills that may come with fevers can be frightening and exhausting. A very high fever can also be dangerous. If the fever is caused by infection, antibiotic medicines will likely be needed.

Some types of chemotherapy or radiation therapy increase the chances of getting infections—usually for a short time following treatments. When treatments reduce the white blood cell count (a condition called "neutropenia"), the person is at a higher risk for infection.

If swelling, pain, redness, or other signs of infection occur, it is important to treat the cause of these problems immediately. Take action before a high temperature develops. The body cannot fight infection well when the white blood cell count is low. Early action is key. If the problem is severe, the doctor may order a medicine to increase the number of white blood cells. Dehydration, which can happen with fever, is also something to be especially alert for since it can become serious and require a trip to the emergency room.

Managing fevers takes organization, and the information in this chapter will help you stay organized. Two topics will be discussed here: coping with fevers and preventing infections.

When to Get Professional Help

Call the doctor, nurse, or the after-hours telephone number <u>right away</u> (no matter what time it is) if any of the following conditions exist:

- *A temperature of 100.5°F or higher, when taken by mouth.* A temperature of 98.6°F is normal for most people, and any temperature above that is a fever. Temperatures of 100.5°F and higher usually indicate a problem requiring medical help. If the person's normal temperature is different from 98.6°F, ask the doctor or nurse what temperature indicates a fever. Usually, two degrees above the person's normal temperature is considered a fever.

Buy a new thermometer if you do not have one you can trust and read easily. A digital thermometer is the easiest to use. It lights up and displays the person's exact temperature. Digital thermometers take the guesswork out of deciding whether a person has a fever. Ask your pharmacist or a store clerk to help you select one. Do not use a rectal thermometer unless your doctor or nurse approves its use. If the person's platelet count is low, the delicate tissue in the rectum may bleed if a thermometer is inserted.

- **Severe shaking chills that last twenty minutes or more.** Chills happen before a person's temperature rises. Take the person's temperature when chills have stopped.
- **Frequent, painful urination.** Pain with urination usually indicates a urinary infection. People with this type of infection may feel the urge to urinate even when there is very little urine in the bladder. When they do urinate, a sharp pain shoots through the lower abdomen, and there may be a burning sensation.
- **No urine output for six to eight hours.** If the person has not urinated in the past six to eight hours, this condition is important to report. This condition has many different possible causes, including infection, and needs to be investigated.
- **New cough, shortness of breath, or rapid breathing.** Report any problems with breathing or coughing, especially any breathing problems. Labored or difficult breathing could be caused by an infection and should be reported, even if the person does not have a fever.
- **Changes in mental status.** Cloudy thinking or mild confusion may be a sign of infection and should be reported.

Some symptoms are not an emergency but should be reported **during regular office hours**. Call your health care provider if any of the following conditions exist:

- **Weakness and inability to drink fluids.** Drinking fluids is important for a person with a fever. When the person's temperature rises, the body loses water that needs to be replaced. If it is not replaced, the person may become dehydrated. Fevers can cause severe fatigue, which makes it hard to drink. If the person has a fever, pay attention to the amount of liquid he or she is able to take in, and report that to the doctor when you call.
- **Any new redness or swelling on the skin or at an IV or injection site.** Skin redness or swelling can indicate an infection. When the white blood cell count is low, small cuts or scrapes can easily become infected.

- **Symptoms of a cold, such as runny nose, stuffy nose, watery eyes, or sore throat.** Infections develop quickly in the mouth or throat. Report cold symptoms, even if there is no fever.
- **New sinus, abdominal, or back pain.** New pain in these areas may be the result of a new infection or the spread of an old infection.
- **Toothache.** Infections in the mouth or gums can cause toothaches. Antibiotics are often prescribed to prevent infection around the tooth. Dental work should be postponed until enough antibiotics are in the bloodstream to fight infection. Check with the doctor treating the infection before scheduling any invasive dental work.
- **Aching and lack of energy that doesn't go away.** These debilitating symptoms may be the result of a low-grade infection.

Have the following information available when you call the doctor or nurse:

- How long has the fever been above 100.5°F? You may not know exactly how long the person has had a fever. Do the best you can to report the time you first took the person's temperature and when you first noticed any other changes, such as redness, sweating, or chills.
- How much liquid did the person with fever drink in the last eight hours or since the fever began, and how much urine has been passed? These measurements tell the doctor or nurse if dehydration is becoming serious.
- Has the person with cancer had other fevers since cancer treatments began? If there has been a pattern of fevers after chemotherapy in the past, provide this information when you call the doctor.
  - How many?
  - When have they occurred?
  - After how many chemotherapy, radiation, or other cancer treatments did they begin?
- What medicines has the person taken to lower the fever or fight infections? Has he or she taken acetaminophen (Tylenol) or antibiotics? When were medicines last taken?
- When was the last cancer treatment, what type was it, and what were the names of any medicines given? Some medicines create mild reactions for a short time. The doctor or nurse can judge what is normal for the medicines that were given.
- What were the person's most recent blood counts, and what date were the blood samples drawn?

What You Can Do

You can manage fevers and infections by following these guidelines:
- **Reduce fever after reporting it.**
- **Prevent fever and infection.**

Reduce Fever After Reporting It

Certain medicines lower fever. These medicines do not solve the problem causing the fever, but they help lower the body temperature and make the person feel better. Encourage the person with cancer to do the following:

➤ **Take acetaminophen unless otherwise directed.**

Acetaminophen lowers body temperature. It also fights swelling and soreness and makes the person more comfortable. Acetaminophen will not solve the problem causing the fever, but it lowers the temperature and reduces side effects of fever, such as fatigue and body aches.

➤ **Take any medicines for fever or infection prescribed by the doctor.**

➤ **Put cold washcloths on the forehead if the person feels hot.**

Cooling the forehead will help reduce the person's discomfort. In addition, the cold washcloths cool the blood that flows through the head close to the surface of the skin, which may help the person feel cooler.

➤ **Drink two to three quarts of cool liquid every twelve hours, unless large amounts of fluid are not allowed.**

When the person is feverish, the body needs more fluid because more fluid than usual is lost through the skin and lungs. A person with a high fever runs the risk of dehydration. Drinking fluids replaces lost water.

➤ **Eat high-calorie, high-carbohydrate foods such as pasta, bread, fruit, potatoes, and energy bars.**

The body's metabolism increases with fever. This increase means that a person with a fever is burning calories at a faster rate than normal. High-calorie, high-carbohydrate foods replace the nutrients that are being used and help restore lost energy.

➤ **Change damp clothing and bed linens.**

The person may get the sweats as the body tries to cool itself down. That moisture will dry on the skin but can leave clothing and bed linens damp and uncomfortable from the person's perspiration. This dampness can also make the body cool down rapidly, causing shaking and chills.

⏩ **Do not overdress the person with a fever.**
Do not pile on blankets or turn up the heat. Overheating the person could increase the fever and thereby cause more problems.

Prevent Fever and Infection

Encourage the person with cancer to do the following to prevent fevers and infections:

⏩ **Wash hands frequently, especially before preparing food, before eating, after using the bathroom, and when tending another sick person, a baby, or a pet.**
Hand washing is the best way to limit the spread of germs. People with cancer can get infections from their own skin, mouth, and tissues. They can also get infections from others. Wash the skin and hands frequently, and brush the teeth at least three times a day to wash away potentially dangerous germs.

⏩ **Use lotions and moisturizers on the skin to keep the skin moist and to prevent drying, chapping, and cracking.**
Bacteria can enter the body through cracks in dry skin and start an infection.

⏩ **Avoid sharing unwashed thermometers, toothbrushes, or drinking glasses.**
Anything that goes in the mouth, including silverware, toothbrushes, and thermometers, can pass germs from one person to another if not washed.

⏩ **Avoid taking rectal temperatures.**
Taking a rectal temperature adds to the risk of infection because the thermometer may cut or injure membranes inside the rectum. If it is not possible to obtain an oral temperature, place the thermometer under the person's armpit. This method is known as taking the axillary temperature.

⏩ **Ask people with colds or other illnesses to postpone visits until they are well.**

⏩ **Avoid raw, unwashed fruits and vegetables, raw or undercooked eggs, and food that has been handled by others when the person's white blood cell count is low.**
People with low white blood cell counts have difficulty warding off infection, and food is a common carrier of germs. Washing (or cooking) fruits and vegetables before eating them removes or destroys many germs. For example, avoid prepared and presliced items, such as presliced meats

and cheeses, prepared salads, and precut fruit. Buy and slice meats, cheeses, fruits, and vegetables at home until white blood cell counts are higher and the risk of infection is lower. See appendix B for information on food safety for people undergoing cancer treatment.

➠ Drink fluids to prevent urinary infections.
Urinary infections are less likely to happen when the kidneys, bladder, and urinary system are flushed with water. Avoid caffeine and alcohol. Drinking about three quarts of liquid each day is recommended.

➠ Practice good dental hygiene, including brushing teeth after eating and soaking dentures daily.
Replace toothbrushes every three months. Toothbrushes harbor bacteria and other organisms because they are wet most of the time. Replace them at least every three months to reduce the chance of infection in the mouth. Also be sure to get a new toothbrush after treating a mouth infection such as a thrush infection.

➠ Thoroughly clean the rectal area after bowel movements.
Women should cleanse the rectal area from front to back to avoid spreading germs to the vagina and opening of the urethra.

➠ Women should use sanitary pads, not tampons, during menstrual periods.
Tampons breed bacteria more easily and can cause tears in the vagina that can lead to infection.

➠ Thoroughly wash skin that is not open to the air, such as the skin in the groin area and underneath the breasts.
Air these areas for a short time after washing to be sure they are dry.

➠ Wear shoes to prevent cuts and bruises.
Even small cuts on the feet can allow bacteria into the body. Cuts do not heal quickly when the white blood cell count is low.

➠ Wash cuts right away with soap and water.
If the person does get a cut, wash it right away.

➠ Use sunscreen, and stay out of the sun between 10:00 a.m. and 4:00 p.m.
Sunburn can lead to blisters that split the skin open. Once the skin is open, it is easier for bacteria to enter the body.

▥➡ **Arrange for someone else to groom pets, empty cat litter boxes, and clean pet cages.**
Pet feces contain many bacteria and fungi, which are easily transferred and can lead to infection in a person with a low white blood cell count. It is best to have someone else clean up after the pets until the person's white blood cell count returns to normal.

Possible Challenges

Consider the following situations that have been difficult for other caregivers:

"He says the fever is just 'burning up' whatever the problem is. He says we don't need to call the doctor."
High fevers are dangerous and should be reported and treated. These conditions can lead to dehydration and seizures. High temperatures do not destroy the bacteria that are causing the problem.

"She says that she's had fevers come and go before, and they didn't last long. She thinks the fever will go away by itself."
If the white blood cell count is low, a fever will not disappear without intervention. Fevers can be serious and should be reported and treated. If the cause of the fever is not treated, the temperature may rise to a dangerous level and the infection can get worse. Report any possible signs of infection, regardless of whether a fever occurs with them.

"We didn't know he had a fever."
If the person's body feels warm or he or she is complaining of aches or other flu-like symptoms, get out the thermometer. Take the person's temperature; if it is above normal, follow the recommendations in this chapter.

Carrying Out and Adjusting Your Plan

Think of other challenges that could interfere with carrying out your plan to manage fevers and infections. What additional roadblocks could get in the way of following the recommendations in this chapter? Will the person with cancer avoid situations that increase risk of infection? Will sick friends and relatives be understanding and willing to postpone their visits? How will you explain your needs to medical professionals? Do you have the time and energy to carry out the plan? Develop plans for getting around these challenges by using the COPE ideas discussed in the introduction.

Keep records of when fevers happen so you can see whether they are occurring more or less frequently. Ensure that the person is avoiding situations that increase risk of infection. If fever remains a problem, or if fevers are happening more often, check the section "When to Get Professional Help" to see whether you need to call the doctor or nurse immediately. If fever continues, ask the doctor or nurse for help. Discuss the results of your plan and what additional steps should be taken to address the problem.

CHAPTER THIRTEEN

Pain

Pain can limit anyone's ability to function and do everyday activities, such as move around, sleep, or eat. Pain also limits one's ability to think clearly. The family caregiver plays an important role in helping the person with cancer manage pain, get relief, and remain comfortable. The caregiver is often the one who administers pain medicines and who makes sure the health care team is informed about the person's response to pain management. The best approach to treat pain is for the caregiver to work with the person with cancer and with the health care team to control and relieve pain. As the caregiver, you need to believe the person's description of his or her pain, assist in reporting it, and assist in following the plan for pain control and relief.

Keep these key ideas in mind as the caregiver of someone with cancer pain:
- *Most cancer pain can be relieved.* All cancer pain can be controlled or managed.
- *Every person with cancer has the right to good pain control and relief.*
- *It takes time to get good pain control and relief.* Have patience, but speak up for the person with cancer.
- *Plans to control and relieve pain need to be reviewed all the time.* Sometimes pain relief plans need to change to work effectively.
- *Reporting pain to health care professionals is absolutely necessary.* Health care professionals and the caregiver must work together to control pain.

Understanding Cancer Pain

Cancer pain has different causes. Like any other pain, it is unpleasant and hurts. Cancer itself can cause pain when it spreads into soft tissue, such as muscle, and when it spreads to organs, such as the liver. Cancer also can spread into the bone or press on a nerve. When it spreads, the cancer causes increased pressure and pain.

Cancer pain also can be caused by medical treatments and procedures. For example, mouth sores can be caused by chemotherapy. Skin irritation or tenderness can be caused by radiation therapy. In addition to cancer pain, a person with cancer also may have serious pain unrelated to the cancer, such as the pain of arthritis.

Types of Pain

There are many sources and types of pain. Pain that arises from bone, joint, muscle, or skin is called *somatic pain* and often is described as aching or throbbing pain. It is easily located because the person can point to where it hurts. Pain that arises from organs such as the stomach, liver, or bowel is called *visceral pain* and may cause cramping pain. It is harder to locate because the person may feel pain all over the abdomen. Pain that arises from nerves is called *neuropathic pain*. Neuropathic pain may be described as burning or shooting pain and usually occurs in certain areas, such as the lower legs or feet, rather than the whole body.

Chronic pain is pain that the person experiences for more than three months. Chronic pain can decrease the person's ability to cope with having cancer and limit the enjoyment of life. If the person has chronic pain, the goal should be to reduce the pain and prevent it from interfering with the person's quality of life. Pain relief measures need to be taken on a regular basis to prevent pain from coming back.

Acute pain is shorter in duration than chronic pain. Acute pain usually is caused by tissue damage. If a person is suffering from acute pain, the goal should be to relieve pain until healing can take place and the pain decreases. Some acute pain may indicate a change in the disease, which requires a change in the treatment plan or immediate medical interventions.

How Pain Is Measured

The first step in dealing with pain is to measure, or assess, the pain. Health care professionals need to understand the cause of the pain so that they can plan the best pain treatment. Doctors and nurses collect information about the person's pain by performing a complete history and physical examination and by reviewing diagnostic tests, such as x-rays, computed tomography (CT) scans, or bone scans. After collecting this information, the doctor will treat the cause of the pain. Treatment can involve surgery, radiation, or medicines to fight cancer. The treatment also will involve medicines to control the pain itself; these medicines are called analgesics. Suggested treatments also include heat, cold, braces, or other methods that do not use medicines.

Health care professionals and people with cancer and their families can use a number of pain assessment tools. Some of these tools are numbered scales (0–10), where 0 indicates no pain and 10 indicates the worst pain there is; some are verbal scales that describe pain with words, such as sharp, burning, or shooting. Other scales use visual images that indicate a person's pain level, such as the FACES rating scale (see figure 13.1). Some cultural groups have designed their own scales with different types of faces, such as certain Native American tribes.

As the caregiver, you must learn how to measure pain, too, so that you can judge whether the pain treatment is working. You can judge the person's pain level by asking him or her to describe the pain or using one of the techniques described on the previous page. Use the same terms or scale each time you ask so you can compare one time with another and monitor changes in the person's pain. For example, the person could choose from the words *worst ever, severe, bad, moderate, mild,* and *none at all* each time, or use the 0–10 scale or FACES scale (see figure 13.1). Another way to measure pain is to think of a 10-inch ruler, where 10 is the worst pain ever, 0 is no pain, and 5 is moderate pain. The person can identify a number on the ruler to match his or her pain. You can use a chart to help keep track of the person's pain level.

Remember that the person with cancer is the only one who can gauge and describe his or her pain. You cannot do this for the person. The person may be experiencing different types of pain and pain in more than one place. For example, someone with cancer may have backaches from arthritis that were there before the cancer. After cancer treatment, he or she might get a new stabbing pain in the hands or feet. After surgery, the person might have sharp pain in the side. All of these types of pain are different and need to be measured and discussed differently.

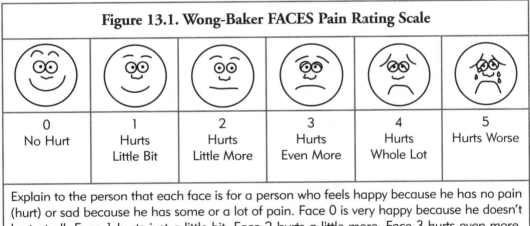

Figure 13.1. Wong-Baker FACES Pain Rating Scale

0 No Hurt	1 Hurts Little Bit	2 Hurts Little More	3 Hurts Even More	4 Hurts Whole Lot	5 Hurts Worse

Explain to the person that each face is for a person who feels happy because he has no pain (hurt) or sad because he has some or a lot of pain. Face 0 is very happy because he doesn't hurt at all. Face 1 hurts just a little bit. Face 2 hurts a little more. Face 3 hurts even more. Face 4 hurts a whole lot. Face 5 hurts as much as you can imagine, although you don't have to be crying to feel this bad. Ask the person to choose the face that best describes how he is feeling. This rating scale is recommended for persons 3 years and older.

From Hockenberry MJ, Wilson D: *Wong's essentials of pediatric nursing,* ed. 8, St. Louis, 2009, Mosby. Used with permission. Copyright Mosby.

When to Get Professional Help

It is important to assess pain often and to report pain levels and any problems controlling pain to the doctor or nurse. Any pain problems should be discussed at each doctor visit. If pain is new or pain relief steps are not working, tell the doctor.

When you call the doctor or nurse, you will want to provide enough information so they can determine whether the person needs to be brought into the emergency room or whether an appointment with the doctor is needed. Often a change in medicines or pain treatment can be made over the phone.

Have the following information available when you call the doctor or nurse:
- When did the pain begin?
- Does the pain come and go or is it constant?
- Where is the pain located? Is it in more than one area?
- Describe the pain:
  - Is the pain sharp and stabbing or dull and aching?
  - Does the pain burn or feel like an electric shock?
  - Is there any numbness or tingling?
  - How severe is the pain? Ask the person to use a number from 0 to 10 to describe or rate the pain, where 0 equals none, 5 equals moderate pain, and 10 equals the worst pain ever experienced. What makes the pain worse? What makes it better?
- How much has this pain interfered with normal activities?
- What has been done to treat the pain? Did this treatment work? How well?
- Has anything interfered with your ability to manage the pain? For example, is the person with cancer afraid of becoming addicted to pain pills, unwilling to take pills on schedule, sleeping through times that pills are scheduled, overdoing physical activities that make the pain worse, not admitting pain, or concerned about the costs of pain medications?
- Describe any medicines used for pain. Name the medicines and doses given, and answer the following questions:
  - How much time elapsed between doses?
  - How many pills have been taken at one time?
  - How many doses were taken in the last two days?
  - How long do they take to work?
  - How much relief do they give?
  - How long does this relief last?
  - What other medicines have been taken or what else has been done to relieve the pain? What were the results?

What You Can Do

There are several things you can do to help manage cancer pain:

- **Understand the pain relief plan.**
- **Understand the types of pain medicines.**
- **Make the best use of pain medicines.**
- **Manage side effects of pain medicines.**
- **Use other methods to prevent or control pain.**
- **Consider complementary therapies as part of the pain relief plan.**

Understand the Pain Relief Plan

You must depend on the doctor to choose the right pain medicine and dosage schedule. Be sure you understand the instructions and the pain relief plan set out by the doctor. The following are three different plans for the use of medicines.

➡ Plan 1: Take medicine as needed ("Give PRN").

Pain medicines can be ordered "as needed," which is sometimes written, "Give prn." For example, if the order says, "Take every three to four hours as needed," the person with pain can take the medicine every three hours and do so consistently, especially if the pain starts to come back three hours after the last dose. Waiting four hours or longer if pain does not return is also okay. Write down the times at which the person takes pain medicine—this information helps the doctor understand how the medicine is working and adjust the prescription and timing to achieve maximum pain relief.

Taking medicine as needed also means the person can take a dose and then wait to take another one until he or she feels the first inkling of pain (as long as that next dose is outside the window of time specified in the doctor's instructions). The person could also take a dose before beginning an activity that stimulates the pain. Some people learn exactly what brings on their pain, such as bending over the stove while cooking or bending over the dryer while doing laundry.

It is usually recommended that the person not take medicines more frequently than ordered. Sometimes taking an extra dose is okay if needed, but check with the doctor first.

➡ Plan 2: Take medicines a certain number of times a day.

If the medicine is prescribed to be taken a certain number of times per day, start with the time the person wakes up and divide the twenty-four hour day into equal spaces. For example, if a doctor orders medicine to be taken twice a day and the person is usually awake at 9:00 a.m., then give a dose at 9:00 a.m. and one at 9:00 p.m. The times do not have to be exact, but try to divide the day into even sections. The person should take medicine during the night if the pain is constant and he or she wakes with pain in the morning. If the person sleeps through the night and is not in severe pain in the morning, you may not have to give the medicine all through the night. Every person's experience with pain is different. Find out what routine works best in your situation. There is some trial and error involved in pain relief.

➤ **Plan 3: Take long-acting medicines every day and give short-acting medicine when needed.**

When pain is chronic and constant, the doctor may order a long-acting medicine, which is typically expected to last eight to twelve hours. It will be prescribed to be taken every eight to twelve hours, every day. If pain is still not controlled on some days (for example, if the person has been particularly active), a short-acting medicine can also be taken. The short-acting medicine may be taken every two hours or every four hours as needed until pain is relieved.

Table 13.1. Pain Diary				
TIME	**PAIN RATING (0–10)**[a]	**NAME OF MEDICINE TAKEN FOR RELIEF**	**SIDE EFFECTS NOTED**[b]	**RATING OF PAIN ONE HOUR AFTER TAKING MEDICATION (0–10)**

[a] Rate pain from 0 to 10, with 0 indicating absence of pain and 10 indicating intense pain.
[b] Did the medicine make the person with cancer drowsy? Did it upset the stomach? What other effect did it cause?

When using this plan in particular, it is a good idea to keep a pain log or diary. Table 13.1 is an example of a pain log using the 0–10 pain scale to rate the pain (0 is no pain, and 10 is the worst pain you can imagine). This will help you keep track of when medicines are taken and the extent to which pain is relieved. If short-term medicine is frequently needed, the long-lasting dose may need to be increased. Discuss frequent use of short-acting medicine with the doctor or nurse.

Understand the Types of Pain Medicines

Almost all cancer pain is treated, at least in part, with medicines. Health care professionals treating cancer pain use a three-step ladder approach developed by the World Health Organization (WHO) for pain relief. The medicinal categories included in the ladder are nonopioid medicines, such as acetaminophen and nonsteroidal anti-inflammatory medicines (NSAIDS); opioids; and adjuvant (additional) medicines.

In the ladder approach, people in pain are assigned to a step in the ladder based on their reports of pain levels. The steps match the intensity of the person's pain. Step 1 is for mild pain, step 2 is for moderate pain, and step 3 is for severe pain.

⫸ Step 1—for mild pain

Medicines recommended in step 1 of the ladder to control mild pain are those for pain rated 1 to 4 on a 10-point scale. They include nonopioid medicines, NSAIDs, and adjuvant medicines.

⫸ Step 2—for moderate pain

Medicines recommended in step 2 of the ladder are meant to control pain rated 5 to 6 on a 10-point scale. If step 1 medicines do not work or the pain is rated as moderate pain, step 2 medicines are used. Medicines recommended in step 2 of the ladder include low-dose opioids and those listed in step 1 (nonopioid medicines, NSAIDs, and adjuvant medicines).

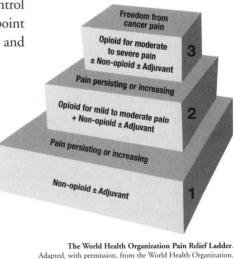

The World Health Organization Pain Relief Ladder.
Adapted, with permission, from the World Health Organization.
http://www.who.int/cancer/palliative/painladder/en/. Accessed June 10, 2011.

⫸ Step 3—for severe pain

Medicines recommended in step 3 of the ladder are meant to control pain rated 7 to 10 on a 10-point scale. If the person with cancer is having severe pain, stronger medicines may be needed. Medicines recommended in step 3 include strong opioids, in addition to NSAIDs and adjuvant medicines.

As a caregiver, you need to learn about the three main classes of pain medicines listed in the ladder: nonopioids (acetaminophen and NSAIDs), opioids, and adjuvant medicines.

Nonopioids

Nonopioids are mild pain relievers. This class includes acetaminophen (Tylenol) and NSAIDs, such as aspirin and ibuprofen (Motrin or Advil). These medicines are used in all steps of the analgesic ladder. NSAIDs are mainly analgesic and anti-inflammatory. Acetaminophen is an analgesic, but it is not an anti-inflammatory medicine. (An analgesic is a drug that relieves pain. An anti-inflammatory is a drug that reduces inflammation, which can cause pain. Some analgesics are anti-inflammatories.) NSAIDs are very effective in treating bone pain caused by cancer, especially when combined with opioids.

NSAIDs have a "ceiling effect," which refers to the dose beyond which no further pain relief will occur. Higher doses will not provide additional pain relief, though side effects will become more severe. NSAIDs do not cause tolerance (physical dependence) or addiction (psychological dependence).

There are different types of NSAIDs. Although NSAIDs work similarly, individual response varies greatly, and so a person who has not responded to one NSAID should try another. Examples of the different NSAIDs are aspirin, ibuprofen, indomethacin, diclofenac, and celecoxib.

Side effects of NSAIDs

The most common side effects of NSAIDs include an increased risk of bleeding caused by reduced platelet aggregation in the blood (decreasing the clotting process); stomach irritation (such as indigestion or burning sensations); and occasional kidney malfunction, especially in the elderly or persons who are dehydrated.

Although selective COX-2 inhibitors (e.g., celecoxib) are NSAIDs, they have different side effects. COX-2 inhibitors cause less stomach irritation than some other medicines and minimal platelet problems, but they may cause cardiac problems. These medicines should be used with caution, especially in people with heart disease.

Overall, acetaminophen is better tolerated than are NSAIDs. It does not cause stomach irritation and does not affect the platelets in the blood; however, it may cause liver failure, especially in people with a history of alcoholism or liver disease. Acetaminophen may cause liver problems if taken at high doses. In adults, the daily dose of acetaminophen should not exceed four grams.

Opioids

Opioids are more powerful than nonopioids and more effective for more intense pain. They are also known as narcotics. Opioids are used for moderate to severe pain in steps 2 and 3 of the analgesic ladder. They are used often for treating cancer pain. Low-dose (step 2) opioids are often combined with acetaminophen. Examples of opioids used in this category are Percocet (which contains oxycodone and acetaminophen), Tylenol with Codeine No. 3 (which contains codeine and acetaminophen), and Lortab (which contains hydrocodone and acetaminophen).

Stronger (step 3) opioids include morphine, hydromorphone, oxycodone, fentanyl, methadone, and oxymorphone. Most opioids are available in two forms: immediate release (short acting) and sustained release (long acting).

People who have constant or frequent pain will benefit from scheduled around-the-clock dosing, which can be easily provided by sustained-release medicines. These medicines stay at a steady level in the plasma and prevent pain from coming back for twenty-four hours. The pain relief effect of sustained-release opioids, such as oral morphine (MS Contin or Oramorph), lasts for eight to twelve hours. Kadian, another form of oral morphine, is a slow-release pill that lasts for up to twenty-four hours. Fentanyl is available as a patch that delivers the drug through the skin continuously for seventy-two hours.

If pain persists in spite of sustained-release medicines, immediate-release medicine can be used as a "rescue" dose. The type of medicine used for breakthrough pain—intensifying pain or pain that flares despite the use of regular medicines—is usually the same as the around-the-clock medicine. Some opioids are not available as sustained-release medicines, and so sometimes two different opioids can be used, one as a long-acting drug and the other as a short-acting drug. Immediate-release opioids work relatively quickly, within ten to thirty minutes of taking the medicine.

When a person cannot swallow tablets or liquid because of swallowing problems, some medicines can be taken by placing them inside the cheek or between the cheek and gums. The medicine is absorbed through the lining of the mouth. This method is called transmucosal administration. An example of this method is the oral transmucosal fentanyl, a lollipop, and the fentanyl effervescent buccal tablet. These forms are absorbed faster than pills, so pain relief happens in five to ten minutes.

Side Effects of Opioids

Side effects caused by opioids include constipation, drowsiness, nausea and vomiting, myoclonus (irregular and involuntary muscle contraction), itching, and delirium (confusion). Constipation is the most common side effect related to opioids. The best way to treat constipation is to be proactive and prevent it. Talk to your doctor about taking a mild laxative and a stool softener on a daily basis. One of the most common regimens includes one or two capsules of the stool softener docusate (Colace) and one or two tablets of senna (a mild laxative) every night. If constipation occurs in spite of following this bowel regimen, a stronger laxative, such as lactulose, can be added. Every person's bowel regimen is unique. A number of laxatives exist that can be combined to better meet each person's needs.

Drowsiness is often experienced at the beginning of opioid treatment and may recur every time the dose is increased. This side effect usually lasts from a few days to a few weeks. It can be relieved by reducing the dose of the drug, changing to another opioid, or taking a psychostimulant (medicine used to treat excessive drowsiness caused by the opioids), such as modafinil (Provigil) or methylphenidate (Ritalin). Such medicines are given in the morning to keep the person awake during the day. They do not interfere with pain relief.

Nausea and vomiting may occur at the beginning of opioid treatment, but these side effects usually subside after a few days or few weeks. Relief may be achieved with the use of antiemetics (drugs used to treat nausea and vomiting), which can be taken around the clock for the first week of treatment with opioids. Examples of antiemetics include prochlorperazine (Compazine), metoclopramide (Reglan), ondansetron (Zofran), and granisetron (Kytril).

Myoclonus is a condition characterized by jerky movements. It may occur when the dose of opioids is too high or has been increased too quickly. To relieve this side effect, the doctor may reduce the dose, change to another opioid, or prescribe a benzodiazepine to treat this symptom. Clonazepam (Klonopin) is the benzodiazepine most commonly used to treat myoclonus.

Itching can occur with any opioid, but this symptom is seen more frequently with morphine. Opioid-induced itching is treated with such antihistamines as diphenhydramine (Benadryl) or hydroxyzine (Atarax). If itching does not subside with antihistamines, the opioid should be changed to one that produces less itching. Fentanyl and oxymorphone both cause less itching.

Delirium is experienced as confusion and occasionally as visual hallucinations. Delirium can occur after the dose of an opioid has been increased. This problem usually goes away after decreasing the dose of the opioid. However, if the dose of opioid cannot be reduced because of pain control, the opioid can be changed to another opioid that does not induce delirium. Delirium can also be treated with a medicine called haloperidol (Haldol).

Make the Best Use of Pain Medicines

Follow these recommendations to make the best use of pain medicines at home:

➡ **Set an alarm as a reminder to administer pain medicine.**

An alarm reminds you to give the pain medicine or reminds the person with cancer to take the medicine.

➡ **Use a medicine tray or pillbox with slots for times of day to hold the medicines.**

Plastic boxes with squares for each day of the week and slots for dose times organize doses. Many people fill the box for the whole week. You can also use an egg carton and mark each slot with the name of the day of the week and the time the pain medicine is to be given that day.

▶ Telephone the pharmacy before going to fill pain prescriptions.

Some pharmacies do not carry all pain medicines. They may have to order it or send you to another store.

▶ Use one pharmacy, if possible.

If you use one pharmacy, the pharmacists will better understand the medicine plan and how it is working. They will share suggestions on how to handle side effects. They will know what pain medicines to keep on hand and can answer many of your questions about the medicines. They will also be able to warn you about possible drug interactions. Drug interactions occur when one drug affects how another drug works.

▶ Keep at least a five-day supply of pain medicine.

Call the doctor for a new prescription before giving the last of any pain medicine. If you are planning to be out of town, be certain to have enough medicine to last until your planned return.

▶ Consider different ways that pain medicine can be taken.

Although most people can take pills for the relief of their chronic pain, there are times when a different way to take medicine is required.

There are many ways to take pain medicines besides pills or tablets:

- **Liquid pain medicines**
  If someone with pain cannot eat solid foods, he or she may have trouble swallowing pills. Liquid medicine may be more easily swallowed.
- **Skin patches**
  A recent advance is the transdermal skin patch, which is placed on the body (chest or back) and delivers medicine through the skin for up to seventy-two hours. For continued pain relief, change the patch every seventy-two hours.
- **Rectal suppositories**
  Pain medicine also comes in rectal suppositories. Once placed in the body, they melt and are absorbed into the bloodstream.
- **Injections**
  Injections (shots) may be given periodically into the subcutaneous tissue (fatty tissue).

The following additional administration methods require some supervision and help from the health care team (though they can be given in the hospital or at home):

- **Subcutaneous (Sub-Q) needles placed under the skin and left there for several days**

  Medicine is administered through the needle every few hours by a family caregiver. These lines can also be hooked to pumps, which deliver the medicine at regular intervals. A nurse will need to move the needle to a new location every few days.

- **IV lines inserted into large veins**

  IV lines inserted into large veins are called "Hickman catheters," "Broviac catheters," or "peripherally inserted central catheters" (PICCs). These catheters are all placed into large veins of the arm. The tubing extends from the skin by a few inches, and medicine is given in a similar way to an IV line. The dressings are changed by nurses at the clinic or at home.

- **Ports implanted under the skin**

  An implanted port is a new way to get medicine into a large vein in the chest. These metal circular ports are about one inch wide and one inch deep. They are usually surgically placed under the skin of the upper chest, and a nurse can find the exact placement by gently pushing on the skin to feel the small round disc. The nurse cleans the skin with a solution and injects medicine into the port, which then flows into the vein. Sometimes the site can be used to draw blood for laboratory tests.

- **IV infusing pumps attached to implanted ports**

  There are also small, portable pumps with IV lines that can be carried on a belt. They run on batteries and deliver medicine evenly throughout the day and night. Home health care nurses can manage these pumps and teach family caregivers how to care for the pump and line. Some people with cancer can give themselves medicine through these lines as well.

- **Epidural catheters near the spine**

  Anesthesiologists can put epidural catheters near the spine to deliver medicines, and family caregivers can be taught how to give medicines through these catheters. A pump can be used to give the medicine continuously.

Manage Side Effects of Pain Medicines

Not all people react the same way to pain medicines, but some side effects are very common. Take measures to prevent side effects and deal with any side effects promptly:

➠ **Prevent constipation with diet, liquids, stool softeners, and laxatives.**
Opioid pain medicines cause constipation by slowing down the bowel, which leads to loss of water from the stool. This loss of water makes the stool hard and difficult to pass. Stool softeners and laxatives can help put water back into the stool, making it softer and easier to pass. People taking opioids are usually placed on bowel management programs to prevent constipation. Ask your doctor or nurse about ways to prevent constipation.

Try a product such as magnesium hydroxide (Milk of Magnesia) if stool softeners and laxatives do not work and the person with cancer has not had a bowel movement in two to three days. You may have to increase the number of stool softeners and stimulants taken every day or give a mild enema. Review the chapter on constipation for additional ways prevent this condition. Encourage the person with cancer to eat foods high in fiber, such as prunes, fresh fruit (except bananas), fresh vegetables, and bran. These foods add bulk to the stool and attract water back into the intestines, which softens the stool. Offer healthy fluids—as many as eight to ten glasses a day. The person should also avoid foods that tend to cause constipation, such as cheese or chocolate.

➠ **Relieve a dry mouth with crushed ice, hard candy, and frequent rinses with water or products that do not contain alcohol.**

➠ **Relieve painful dry nasal passages by humidifying the air or breathing in warm moisture from a sink full of warm water.**
Saline drops or saline nasal sprays (such as Ocean) may be purchased at a pharmacy, and both are helpful.

➠ **Avoid an upset stomach by taking medicine with food, unless instructed to do otherwise by the pharmacist or physician.**
Some pain medicines can cause stomach upset if taken on an empty stomach.

➠ **Relieve mild itching by gently rubbing the area with a cool damp cloth.**
Mild itching may occur for a few days. You can use a cloth dipped in cool water to soothe the itching.

➠ **Catch up on sleep once pain is relieved.**
If sleepiness increases just after starting or increasing pain medicine, wait about three days before getting overly concerned. Sometimes sleepiness happens because a person is finally getting pain relief and needs to catch up on missed rest or because the body needs time to adjust to new medicines or doses. If sleepiness is a concern, offer beverages with caffeine in them, if allowed by the doctor. Discourage driving a car or operating power tools since opioids slow response time.

Use Other Methods to Prevent or Control Pain

Consider using the following ideas in your pain relief plan:

➡ Use warm showers, warm baths, hot water bottles, or warm washcloths.
Heat relaxes the muscles and gives a sense of comfort. Do not set heating pads on high because they can burn the skin. Do not place heating pads over or near radiation marks on the skin, even after radiation treatments are finished. If the person is wearing a patch that provides pain medicine, do not place heat on the patch since heat can increase the amount of medicine released from the patch.

➡ Use cool cloths or ice.
Cooling the skin and muscles can soothe pain, especially pain that comes from inflammation or swelling. For example, many people like using a cool washcloth on their foreheads when they have a headache.

➡ Position the person carefully with pillows and soft seat cushions.

➡ Massage sore spots, such as the neck and shoulders.

➡ Practice deep breathing exercises.
Breathing deeply, slowly, and quietly helps the mind and body to relax, which helps decrease pain. Use voice recordings or follow instructions in books on relaxation. Ask the health care team for recommendations, or read the chapter on anxiety to learn more about relaxation techniques.

➡ Plan pleasant, involving activities.
Activity can help take one's mind off the pain. Different people are distracted by different activities. One person may be distracted by watching television or looking at a catalog. Another may be distracted by listening to music or visiting with friends. Plan activities during times when the person with pain is feeling best and is most alert.

➡ Ask for help with tasks.
Now is the time for both you and the person with cancer to get others to lend a hand. Don't be shy about asking for help! It is part of your job as a caregiver to get help when you need it.

➡ Use prayer or meditation to cope with pain.

➠ **Avoid stressful events when possible.**

Emotional stress and anxiety increase awareness and sensitivity to pain. If you can cancel or avoid stressful events, do so. See the chapters on anxiety and depression for ways to control emotional stress.

➠ **Encourage the person to attend a support group meeting for people with cancer or an educational session.**

Many people with cancer enjoy these meetings, and family and friends are welcome. To find out where and when local support groups meet, call your American Cancer Society at **800-227-2345** or look online or in the telephone book. You can also ask nurses, doctors, or social workers at your hospital about support groups in your area.

Consider Complementary Therapies as Part of the Pain Relief Plan

Complementary therapies can also be part of an effective pain relief plan. Complementary therapies are supportive methods that are used in addition to conventional treatments. Complementary therapy can include massage therapy, meditation, yoga, art therapy, and many other approaches, in addition to more common supportive approaches such as psychological therapy and physical therapy.

You may need to ask for a referral from the doctor to someone who can provide these treatments. For more information on complementary therapies, visit **cancer.org** or look at the resource guide at the end of this book.

➠ **Consider psychological approaches.**

Examples of psychological approaches for pain relief are contingency relief, cognitive behavioral therapy, biofeedback, relaxation, hypnosis, and psychotherapy. Contingency relief includes methods to help people change their behavior associated with pain. Cognitive behavioral therapy helps people change their perceptions of pain, increase their sense of control, and reduce maladaptive behaviors. Biofeedback teaches people how to take control of their body responses. Relaxation reduces a person's focus on pain, muscle tension, and emotional arousal. Hypnosis uses the person's susceptibility to suggestion to modify memory and perception of pain. Psychotherapy can be used to treat depression or anxiety associated with chronic pain. It helps modify symptoms, change maladaptive behaviors, and promote personal growth.

➠ **Consider physical rehabilitative approaches.**

Physical rehabilitative interventions can be quite beneficial to people with chronic pain. These interventions relieve pain, improve physical function, improve energy levels, and alter physiological responses to pain. Some examples include physical therapy, exercise, stretching, and gait and posture training. Other physical therapies for pain include thermotherapy (the use of heat), cryotherapy (the use of cold), and electroanalgesia (the use of transcutaneous electrical nerve stimulation [TENS] to reduce pain).

⠿➡ Radiopharmaceuticals, radiation therapy, and pain clinics

Some types of pain may require additional and less common medical interventions.

- ***Radiopharmaceuticals***

    These are radioactive medicines used to treat pain caused by bone metastasis. A therapeutic dose of the medicine is given intravenously once only. Benefits can be observed two to three weeks after its administration. However, before the pain is relieved, people may experience an increase in pain for a few days. The main side effect is a decrease in the blood cell count.

- ***Radiation therapy***

    Sometimes radiation therapy is prescribed to shrink a tumor that is causing pain. Treatments usually are given daily for a period of a few days up to four to five weeks.

- ***Pain clinics***

    Some universities and large hospitals have special clinics to evaluate and treat chronic pain. Most pain clinics require that patients come to them through a doctor's referral. If chronic pain is not being managed effectively, ask the doctor about seeing a specialist in pain relief. There may be a pain clinic at your hospital, or you may have to be referred to a different hospital. Specialists at pain clinics know a lot about special procedures for managing pain. For example, an anesthesiologist can give a nerve block to stop pain for a short time until other methods can be prescribed, or the nerve block can be given to last a long time. Another advantage of a pain clinic is the staff might prescribe a combination of two or three medicines that relieve different types of pain.

Possible Challenges

Consider the following situations that have been difficult for other caregivers:

"I'm afraid of addiction."

People who take opioids for cancer pain do not become addicted. In fact, if their pain is treated effectively, it decreases the risk of addiction. People who are addicts take medicines for a high or an altered state of mind. People who take opioids for cancer pain take them to get relief from physical pain. People who are not addicts before they take opioids for cancer pain do not become addicts later. Remember the medicine is being used for pain control and not for a psychological high. Even if you know that your friend or family member is not addicted, others may not. Tell them this medicine is part of the medical treatment and absolutely crucial to the person's quality of life.

"I want to save the pain medicine for when the pain is severe."

Taking pain medicine for mild discomfort now does not affect how well it will work when the pain gets worse. Don't refrain from taking pain medicines in order to save up for later. In reality, it takes more medicine to treat pain that hasn't been controlled than it does to prevent pain from worsening. People sometimes need to increase their doses of pain medicine. The need for more medicine does not mean they are becoming "immune" to pain medicines or that their tolerance for the medicine has changed. These people need more medicine or different combinations of medicine because the pain has changed. If the person reaches the dose limit for a particular medicine, the doctor can change to a different medicine. Also, taking enough medicine now helps the person with pain relax and preserve his or her strength. Keeping pain under control is important for the person's peace of mind.

"No one wants to hear about my pain."

Family and friends may seem uninterested because they feel helpless. Doctors and nurses who specialize in pain, such as those in a pain clinic or hospice, do understand pain problems. Talk to them if you are feeling alone with these problems.

"He doesn't want to take any morphine because he thinks that means he's dying. Only people who are close to death take morphine."

Morphine is not reserved for the dying. It is an effective medicine for many types of cancer pain. Taking it does not mean a person is near death. It is used to control chronic pain for patients in many different types of situations. Some people are able to return to work and resume their regular daily activities because morphine is so effective in relieving their pain. It lets them return to pain-free lives.

Carrying Out and Adjusting Your Plan

Think of other challenges that could interfere with carrying out your plan to manage pain. What additional roadblocks could get in the way of following the recommendations in this chapter? Will the person with cancer take the necessary pain medicine? What methods of taking the medicine will be most effective? How will you measure the person's pain? How will you explain your needs to medical professionals? Do you have the time and energy to carry out the plan? Develop plans for getting around these challenges by using the COPE problem-solving steps in the introduction.

Pain control can be a process of trial and error, but it is possible to control the person's pain. You, the person with cancer, and the health care team will need to work together to find a pain relief plan that works. It may require flexibility and patience, but pain control is obtainable. Communication is very important. One way to communicate with physicians and nurses is to speak the same language—share the same vocabulary and understanding about pain. You now have some information that will help you understand what the health care provider is talking about, for example, when he or she orders an opioid analgesic. If you are not sure your plan is effective or have questions, share your concerns with the health care provider.

CHAPTER FOURTEEN

Mouth Problems

Problems with the mouth are a common side effect of cancer treatments. The skin inside the mouth contains rapidly growing cells. Chemotherapy can damage the healthy cells in the mouth, weakening the mouth tissues. Mouth sores can develop (a condition known as mucositis or stomatitis), and these sores take longer to heal than they would in a person not undergoing chemotherapy. Mouth problems associated with cancer treatments can be very painful and can interfere with eating.

Cancer and cancer treatments can temporarily reduce the person's ability to fight infection. When the immune system cannot protect the body from normal bacteria or outside germs, weakened or inflamed tissues in the mouth can become infected. A sore and tender throat and esophagus (the tube leading to the stomach) can also develop.

When to Get Professional Help

Health care professionals can determine whether the mouth, tongue, throat, or esophagus is becoming infected. Sometimes mouth problems become so severe that the person must take pain medication or be hospitalized for antibiotic therapy.

Call the doctor or nurse if any of the following conditions exist:

- *Temperature rises to more than 100.5°F.* Fever can indicate a mouth infection. If the person's temperature goes up suddenly, report it. Remember, however, that a mouth infection can occur before the temperature goes up, so fever is not the only indication of an infection.
- *Slight redness in the mouth gets much redder.* The skin in the mouth will turn red before a mouth sore develops. You will need a light to tell whether the mouth, gums, or tongue is redder than usual. Use a small flashlight to look into the mouth for redness or

sores. Check the mouth twice a day, morning and night. Look at the roof of the mouth and inspect the gums and under the tongue. If the person wears dentures, remove them before checking the mouth.

- **Redness on the tongue turns to white patches, or white patches appear on gums or elsewhere in the mouth.** White patches indicate infection. Usually, it is a thrush infection (caused by the fungus *Candida albicans*). This infection occurs when the lining in the mouth is unable to fight off normal bacteria, and bacteria increase in number and become a problem.

- **The person complains of "cotton mouth" or a very thick feeling on the tongue when rubbed against the upper teeth.** A cottony feeling in the mouth or on the tongue may mean an infection is starting. Call and report this symptom right away.

- **A sore or an ulcer appears on the lips or in the mouth.** If the skin in the mouth is affected by chemotherapy, mouth soreness and sometimes mouth sores or ulcers follow.

- **The person has a sore or painful throat.** The lining of the throat is made up of the same type of cells as the lining of the mouth. The throat is just as likely as the mouth to get red and sore.

- **Difficulty in swallowing prevents the person from taking medicine as often as prescribed.** Trouble with swallowing can cause problems taking medicine. When the throat is sore or swollen, swallowing becomes more difficult. Call the doctor if medicines are skipped because swallowing is too painful.

- **The person has been unable to take in much food or fluid for two days.** Difficulty in swallowing can make it difficult to eat or drink. The person with cancer may be eating or drinking less because of a sore or painful throat. Lack of food and water can cause weakness and dehydration. Treatment can ease the pain associated with eating and drinking.

Have the following information available when you call the doctor or nurse:

- When did the mouth problems start?
- Is the mouth, tongue, or throat redder than usual?
- Are there white patches in the mouth?
- What foods and beverages has the person consumed in the past forty-eight hours?
- How are the mouth and teeth cleaned? Are any special rinses used to prevent mouth sores?
- Is the person with cancer smoking or using an oral tobacco product? If yes, how much?
- Was any alcohol consumed? If yes, how much?
- Have there been changes in the person's ability to chew or swallow?
- Has any medicine been ordered for the mouth or throat? If so, how often is it taken?

- Do any medicines for the mouth cause problems, such as gagging or nausea, that result in their being taken less frequently than prescribed?
- When was the last radiation or chemotherapy treatment, and what chemotherapy medicines were given? Have there been any recent changes in treatments?
- Is the person taking any medications, including herbs or vitamins, not prescribed by a doctor?

What You Can Do

There are several things you can do to deal with mouth sores or a sore mouth:

- **Moisten a dry mouth.**
- **Soothe a sore mouth and ease swallowing.**
- **Treat mouth sores, ulcers, and infections.**
- **Prevent mouth sores.**

Moisten a Dry Mouth

Dry mouth is a frequent side effect of medicines taken for cancer and makes it harder to chew and swallow. There are several ways to help a dry mouth. Encourage the person with a dry mouth to do the following:

➡ **Rinse the mouth with water before meals and throughout the day.**
Rinsing the mouth with water helps to moisten it and remove the feeling of being parched or dry. Don't use mouthwashes that have alcohol in them—they dry the mouth.

➡ **Use a lip moisturizer before eating.**
If the lips are moist, food is easier to chew and enjoy. Put a thin coat of petroleum jelly, lip salve, or cocoa butter on the lips.

➡ **Drink small sips of liquids with meals.**

➡ **Sip two to three quarts of liquid a day, unless large amounts of fluid are not allowed.**

➡ **Eat ice chips, Popsicles, frozen juices, or frozen drinks.**
These frozen liquids are hydrating and refreshing. The sugar content in Popsicles also makes the mouth water, which decreases dryness.

⟶ **Dunk bread, crackers, and baked foods in coffee, tea, milk, or soup to make them moist.**
Moistening food makes it easier to chew and swallow. Dip bread in soup, shredded meat in marinades or sauces, or toast in coffee.

⟶ **Mix gravies, sauces, salad dressings, melted butter or margarine, mayonnaise, or yogurt into food.**
Sauces and gravies are good ways to moisten food. They can be added toward the end of cooking or when food is reheated.

⟶ **Eat soft, liquid foods.**
These foods include applesauce, canned fruits, casseroles, cooked cereal, baby foods, Popsicles, custard, cottage cheese, bananas, puddings, ice cream, gelatin, sherbet, yogurt, milk shakes, soups, stews, watermelon, and seedless grapes. Solid foods can be ground or put in the blender. Many people with cancer use blenders to prepare foods they cannot chew easily. Even a steak can be tenderized and puréed, and all of the good flavor remains.

⟶ **Ask about artificial saliva.**
Artificial saliva can be ordered through most pharmacies. It comes in a bottle and is made of glycerin, purified water, and a few other ingredients. MouthKote and Salivart are examples of commercial products that are available in a mint flavor. Gum products, such as Biotene gum, can help stimulate saliva.

Soothe a Sore Mouth and Ease Swallowing

Some types of chemotherapy cause mouth sores, which make eating and swallowing difficult. Encourage the person with cancer to do the following to soothe a sore mouth and ease swallowing:

⟶ **Rinse the mouth with a baking soda solution after eating.**
Prepare a solution of ½ teaspoon of baking soda in 1 cup of tap water. Solutions of salt, baking soda, or both mixed with water (see recipes on page 149) soothe the mouth and help it heal. Rinsing the mouth after eating removes food particles that could irritate the gums. These homemade solutions are more gentle than commercial mouthwashes, many of which contain alcohol.

⟶ **Avoid using mouthwashes with alcohol in them.**
Many mouthwashes have alcohol in them and can sting and dry the mouth. Commercial

mouthwashes that do not contain alcohol are gaining in popularity and are available at any pharmacy. Ask a pharmacist for assistance to find one.

IIII➡ **Drink plenty of liquids and suck on ice chips.**

IIII➡ **Use a blender or hand masher to soften foods.**
Softer foods are easier to chew and swallow. They are less likely to tear any sores or scrape raw tissues.

IIII➡ **Moisten food with gravy, butter, cream, cottage cheese, ricotta cheese, milk, and sauces.**
Moist food is easier to swallow, especially when the mouth and throat are tender.

IIII➡ **Purée food, and drink it from a cup or through a straw.**
Soft food can be liquefied in a blender and poured into a cup for drinking. Using a straw helps the liquid bypass sore mouth tissues. Many proteins and calories can be taken in this way. If the person is too weak to use a straw, then fill the straw with an inch or two of liquid and drop the liquid in the mouth slowly.

IIII➡ **Eat soft, moist foods that ease swallowing:**
- **Meats and proteins**
  Beef, pork, chicken, and fish should be well cooked, tender, and easy to chew. Other soft forms of protein include smooth peanut butter, eggs, quiche, baby foods, cottage cheese, ricotta cheese, tofu, tempeh, mild cheese, macaroni and cheese, yogurt, and bean casseroles. Avoid sharp cheese, crunchy peanut butter, and spicy foods.
- **Vegetables**
  Include well-cooked vegetables that are easy to chew and baked or mashed potatoes. Avoid vegetables with a lot of acid (such as tomatoes and tomato soups or sauces), potato skins, crunchy or raw vegetables, and fried potatoes or vegetables.
- **Fruits**
  Applesauce, apple juice, grape juice, nectars, prune juice, soft cooked or fresh noncitrus fruits, and bananas are good choices. Avoid citrus fruits and their juices, such as oranges, lemons, and grapefruits. These fruits contain acid that will make mouth sores hurt more.
- **Dairy**
  Milk, milk shakes, cream soups, eggnog, buttermilk, custards, and puddings can be included in the diet.

- **Breads**

  Include all cooked or dry soft cereals, soft bread and rolls, and pasta with mild sauce. Avoid seeded breads, crusty breads, or granola bars. Breads and cereals can be softened with milk or other liquids.

▬➡ **Eat foods at room temperature.**

Avoid extremely hot foods.

▬➡ **Let carbonation or fizz escape from sodas.**

Bubbles from carbonation can irritate the mouth or hurt mouth sores.

▬➡ **Eat gelatin, pudding, sherbets, softened ice cream, and Popsicles.**

These foods count as liquids. They are important because the person with mouth sores needs fluids to combat a dry, sore mouth and throat and to prevent dehydration and imbalances of important body chemistry.

▬➡ **Ask about high-calorie liquids, such as Ensure, Isocal, or milk shakes.**

Talk to the health care team about drinking these high-calorie drinks in between meals or after meals.

▬➡ **Ask the doctor about using a numbing liquid as a "throat coat" before eating and swallowing.**

Many people swallow mouth gels or "throat coats" (a thick jelly-like liquid) before meals and at bedtime if the mouth or throat is very sore. This medicine numbs the tongue and throat enough to let liquid and soft foods pass without much trouble. The medicine also usually contains an antacid and an antihistamine, which soothe the soreness and decrease swelling and inflammation, especially in the throat and esophagus. Ask the doctor about these mouth gels or numbing medicines if they haven't been prescribed as part of chemotherapy. If the person has trouble swallowing, speak to the doctor or pharmacist about other medicines for this purpose. There may be other types of soothing medications that are easier for the person to take, such as tablets or lozenges.

▬➡ **Use a topical ointment on mouth sores to soothe pain or soreness.**

Some mouth sores cause so much pain they prevent the person from eating and chewing. Coating the sores with a topical ointment, such as Ambesol, can relieve pain for a while.

➠ **Ask about using mild pain pills.**

Mild pain medicines can be taken an hour before eating and drinking. They help reduce the pain of biting, chewing, or swallowing when the mouth feels sore or there are mouth ulcers.

Treat Mouth Sores, Ulcers, and Infections

Follow these recommendations at the first hint of a problem to reduce the seriousness of a mouth sore or mouth or throat infection.

➠ **Rinse the mouth with warm tap water after eating or drinking, or use any of the following solutions:**
- one-half teaspoon of salt in two cups of water
- one-half teaspoon of baking soda in one cup of water
- one-half teaspoon of salt and one-half teaspoon of baking soda in two cups of water
- three ounces of unsweetened cranberry juice and three ounces of water

Mouth rinses remove food particles that may build up and cause bacteria to grow. Rinses also soothe sore tissues and help them heal faster. Rinse at least four times a day and as often as every two hours while awake, if possible. If the salt rinse burns, use the baking soda recipe or use less salt.

➠ **Ask the doctor about prescription mouth rinses to swish and swallow.**

During chemotherapy and for a few weeks after treatment, many people use a prescription mouth rinse to swish and swallow at least four times per day. This rinse prevents infection and eases soreness.

➠ **Finish any liquid antibiotics when they are prescribed to treat infection.**

The doctor may order an oral liquid antibiotic to kill infection. If the antibiotic is effective, the person's mouth should feel better, and eating and drinking should be easier in a few days. Be sure that the person takes the full course of antibiotics and does not stop taking the medicine when the mouth feels better.

➠ **Avoid using peroxide or peroxide rinses.**

Peroxide kills bacteria, but it also causes drying and can actually lead to a mouth and throat infection known as thrush. In rare cases, a peroxide rinse may be ordered to cleanse a deep sore that is not healing. If prescribed, it should not be used more frequently than instructed. Do not continue using peroxide longer than seven days. If you are uncertain about the use of peroxide, talk with the doctor or nurse. Recent research strongly advises against its use.

➠ **Avoid glycerin swabs.**

Glycerin swabs are drying to the mucous membranes.

➠ **Avoid cigarettes, pipes, chewing tobacco, and alcoholic beverages.**

These will all make mouth sores worse.

Prevent Mouth Sores

Encourage the person with cancer to do the following to prevent mouth sores:

➠ **Brush teeth at least every four hours.**

Try to rinse the mouth every two hours with a salt water or baking soda rinse (see page 149 for a recipe). Rinsing, even with warm water, removes bacteria and food buildup that can lead to mouth infections and sores. Every four hours, try to use any of these methods to clean the teeth: soft toothbrush, soft sponge applicator, cotton tipped applicator, and/or a finger wrapped with gauze or soft washcloth. The mouth can be easily irritated. Softer toothbrushes prevent cutting or scraping and reduce the likelihood of infection.

➠ **Throw away toothbrushes after a mouth infection.**

As a rule, change toothbrushes at least every two months, even if the person has not had any mouth infections. Replace toothbrushes after infections, as toothbrushes can harbor bacteria and start new infections.

➠ **Remove dentures when cleaning the mouth.**

Clean dentures with a toothbrush and a cleansing agent such as Peridex. Rinse dentures with salt water or plain water after cleaning.

➠ **Remove dentures when rinsing or sleeping.**

Dentures can irritate a dry mouth. They also can cause enough scraping to break the skin and start an infection, especially if they don't fit well.

➠ **Keep lips moist with a light coating of petroleum jelly, mild lip balm, or cocoa butter.**

If swallowing is difficult, then the mouth and lips become dry. Lip balms prevent chapping and infection.

➠ **Drink about two to three quarts of fluid each day—unless otherwise directed.**

‣ **Chew sugarless gum or use sugarless hard candies, which moisten the mouth.**
Sugarless gum and candies increase saliva in the mouth. Sugarless products are recommended because they limit the buildup of bacteria. Taking frequent sips of water also helps. Many people carry large plastic cups with straws and drink frequently to keep the mouth moist.

‣ **If the person uses a WaterPik (a dental cleaning device that produces a powerful water jet), use it only on the lowest setting.**
Water from a WaterPik can cause bleeding. The gums may become very sensitive as a side effect of some chemotherapy regimens, and sensitive gums bleed easily.

‣ **Use dental floss at bedtime.**
Flossing removes food particles but can also cause small cuts. These heal during the night because no food is eaten for at least eight or ten hours. Avoid flossing, however, when platelet or white blood cell counts are low, when flossing could cause bleeding or infections. Do not floss if it causes bleeding or pain.

‣ **Avoid commercial mouthwashes that contain alcohol.**
Many commercial mouthwashes have alcohol in them, which causes drying. Ask the nurse for mouthwash recommendations, find an alcohol-free mouthwash, or use the recipes for homemade mouthwashes on page 149.

‣ **Avoid glycerin or lemon juice mouth swabs.**
These products also cause drying. Avoid using them because the skin inside the mouth can crack and become infected when it's dry.

Possible Challenges

Consider the following situations that have been difficult for other caregivers.

"He doesn't want to quit smoking or drinking."
Both smoking and drinking irritate the mouth. If the person is undergoing chemotherapy and doesn't quit either habit, then it's even more important to do other things to take care of the mouth, such as frequent rinsing.

"It's upsetting for him to have soft or mashed foods."
Serve soft foods attractively. Add flavorings that the person likes. Encourage everyone in the family to eat the same or similar foods.

Carrying Out and Adjusting Your Plan

Think of other challenges that could interfere with carrying out your plan to manage mouth problems. What additional roadblocks could get in the way of following the recommendations in this chapter? Will the person with cancer practice good oral hygiene? Will other people help with food preparation? How will you explain your needs to medical professionals? Do you have the time and energy to carry out the plan? Develop plans for getting around these challenges by using the COPE ideas discussed in the introduction.

The most important thing you can do is to set up and follow a regular daily schedule for treating and preventing mouth sores. Check the mouth regularly to spot new or worsening sores. Pay special attention to whether mouth sores interfere with eating, drinking, or taking medicines as directed. If problems with mouth soreness or swallowing are getting worse, review this chapter and ask yourself whether you are doing everything you can to encourage good oral hygiene and to protect the mouth and throat against soreness and infection. Call the doctor or nurse to discuss the results of your plan and what additional steps could be taken to manage the problem.

CHAPTER FIFTEEN

Skin Problems

Skin problems are not usually an emergency, unless they are related to an allergic response to a drug. They can be upsetting and uncomfortable, however, and can indicate other medical problems. As a caregiver, you can help by noticing early signs of skin problems, by helping to treat them, and by encouraging the person with cancer to care for his or her skin.

Many people experience changes in their skin during cancer treatments. Sometimes chemotherapy causes skin changes, some of which are more bothersome than others. The skin can become dry and itchy. Rashes or little sores can appear. Some people sweat more when undergoing chemotherapy. Skin, veins, and fingernails may become darker. Chemotherapy can make the person more prone to sunburn.

Radiation therapy causes skin problems that can last several weeks after treatments are completed. Typical skin reactions include dryness, itching, and redness. These reactions are confined to the skin over the area being treated by radiation. Most skin reactions are mild and go away a few weeks after treatment is finished, but sometimes the treated skin stays dark long after treatment is over.

Some targeted therapies can cause skin changes. The most common skin change is a rash that looks like acne. Other possible changes include dry skin; itching; a feeling like sunburn; red, sore cuticles; burning, dry, or red eyes; changes in the eyelids, such as tenderness, swelling, or crustiness; sores on the scalp; and a condition called hand-foot syndrome, in which the soles of the feet and the palms of the hands become painful and swollen.

Some of the skin problems associated with cancer treatment can be eliminated, some can be reduced, and some will not get better until treatments are completed. Almost all skin problems improve after treatments are over.

When to Get Professional Help

Call the doctor or nurse if any of the following conditions exist:

- *Skin gets very rough, red, or painful.* Roughness or redness may signal an allergic reaction to a new medicine, or the cause could be external, such as an allergic reaction to a detergent, soap, or new food. Be sure to report any changes in the person's treatment regimen (for example, if chemotherapy was started recently, if the dose was changed, or if new medicines were added), as well as any new lotions or soaps the person has used or new foods he or she has eaten.

- *A cut becomes very red, sore, or swollen.* Report any cuts that are not healing. They may be painful to the touch, and the skin around the cut may become shiny, red, and raised. If you act early, you can prevent serious skin infections.

- *Pus comes out of an opening or cut.* Pus usually indicates a skin infection. Pus from any opening should be reported.

- *The feet and/or hands become sore, swollen, or blisters develop.* These could be early symptoms of hand-foot syndrome, and treating it early can help keep it from getting worse.

- *The area around the fingernails or toenails becomes sore or red.* Creams and soaks can help with this problem, but the health care team needs to be sure the area does not get infected.

- *Sores develop on the scalp or other areas with hair.* These should be treated to help prevent scars that could block hair growth later.

- *The eyes get very dry, red, or tender, or eyelashes begin to grow inward toward the eyeball.* This can be a side effect of some targeted therapies, and your health care team can help to manage these conditions.

- *A rash or hives start.* Rashes are areas of red skin, often appearing in unequal blotches that become more red when scratched. Hives are an outbreak of swollen bumps (red or lighter pink in color) that come on suddenly. Hives can sometimes look like welts or long, thin stripes. Rashes or hives could be caused by a drug reaction, a reaction to a food or beverage, or clothing drawn too tightly over a dressing. If you do not know what caused the skin problem and the person has no history of rashes or hives, it's best to call the doctor.

- *Severe itching lasts more than three days.* Itching can be a side effect of some drugs. It can also be caused by the release of chemicals that the body cannot process through the skin—the excess substances get pushed through the pores of the skin.

- *Skin is scratched open and looks red.* If itching becomes severe, the person may scratch the skin raw without even realizing it. Open skin can become infected.

- *Skin turns yellow.* Color changes in the skin can signal organ problems. For example, if a person turns yellow, this change can mean the liver is not working correctly.

- *A bruise does not improve in a week.* Bruises that do not heal can mean that platelet counts are low, and very slow bleeding may still be occurring at the site of the bruise.

Have the following information available before you call the doctor or nurse. This information will help the doctor or nurse determine the seriousness of the skin problems and what to do about them.

- When did the problem start?
- What do you think brought it on?
- How bad or embarrassing is it to the person?
- What helps it feel or look better?
- What is the person's temperature?
- How long does it take for a bruise to go away?
- If there is a rash, when does it appear and when does it go away?
- Are there any cuts that are not healing?
- If there is itching, where is it and what relieves it?
- When was the last chemotherapy treatment?
- What other medicines are being taken and at what doses?
- When was the last radiation treatment and to what area of the body?

What You Can Do

You can manage skin problems by following these guidelines:

- **Prevent dryness and itching.**
- **Relieve itching when it occurs.**
- **Take steps to manage hand-foot syndrome.**
- **Help conceal dark skin, veins, or discolored fingernails.**
- **Treat acne.**
- **Limit sweating.**
- **Limit sun exposure.**
- **Take care of skin during and after radiation therapy.**

Prevent Dryness and Itching

Dryness leads to itching. Both can break skin tissues to the point of cracking open. Encourage the person to take the following steps to prevent or treat dry skin:

▪▪▪▶ Bathe with cool or lukewarm (not hot) water.

Hot water can damage and dry out skin tissues.

➠ **Use gentle soaps or bath oils that do not contain alcohol, perfume, or dyes.**
Harsh soaps are drying and should be avoided. Try an oatmeal soap or a bath oil such as Alpha Keri, which can be added to bath water. You can also add mineral oil or baby oil to bath water. The oil soaks in and prevents the water from drying out the skin; however, be careful since it can make the tub slippery. Put a rubber mat in the tub to prevent falls.

➠ **Take sponge baths instead of full baths or showers.**
Sponge baths are cooler and decrease the amount of time the skin is immersed in water, making them less drying.

➠ **Use premoistened towelettes for bathing.**
Consider using premoistened towelettes that can be placed in the microwave. These towelettes contain a warm cleansing/moisturizing liquid that does not need to be rinsed off. They come in a hand towel size or a larger bath towel size.

➠ **Do not scrub the skin.**
Scrubbing pulls on delicate skin tissues and removes important moisture.

➠ **Rinse skin thoroughly after bathing and pat skin dry.**
Patting is more gentle than rubbing and helps lock in needed moisture.

➠ **Moisturize your skin two times a day with a cream that contains no alcohol, perfume, or dyes.**
The best time to do this is right after bathing, when the skill is still moist.

➠ **Limit bathing to once a day or less.**
Bathing more than once a day leads to excessive dryness because the skin is rubbed and exposed to soap and hot water.

➠ **Drink two quarts (eight glasses) of fluid every day, unless otherwise instructed.**
Drinking fluids reduces the risk of dehydration and restores moisture to skin tissues.

➠ **Avoid extreme heat, cold, or wind.**
Heat, cold, and wind chafe the skin, damaging it as well as drying it out.

➠ **Avoid colognes, aftershaves, or after-bath splashes that contain alcohol.**
These products dry the skin.

‖‖➡ **Use an electric razor.**

Electric razors are less likely than razor blades to scrape off layers of skin.

‖‖➡ **Avoid opening or popping blisters, and put dry, clean gauze on any open areas.**

‖‖➡ **Wash sheets, towels, and clothing in gentle laundry soap.**

Harsh detergents that attack oil or stains have more chemicals that are irritating to tender skin. Harsh detergents can remain on clothes, towels, and sheets and can cause itching and irritation.

‖‖➡ **Keep rooms cooled to between 60° and 70°F.**

Keep the house, particularly the person's bedroom, at a comfortable, cool temperature. Sweating increases itchiness.

‖‖➡ **Cover up in the sun.**

Heat from the sun causes sweating, which will increase itching. Covering up also prevents sunburn and drying of the skin. If you will be outside during the day, use a sunscreen with an SPF of at least 30 that contains zinc oxide or titanium oxide at least one to two hours before going out.

Relieve Itching When It Occurs

Encourage the person with cancer to take the following steps to relieve itching:

‖‖➡ **Add baking soda to bath water.**

Baking soda soothes sensitive skin and decreases itching. You can also try an oatmeal bath. Products are also available in drug stores that can help to relieve itching.

‖‖➡ **Apply cool, moist compresses to itchy areas.**

Cool soaks are soothing and relieve itching, at least for a short time. Use washcloths or soft dish towels soaked in cool water and wrung out.

‖‖➡ **Keep nails short and clean.**

Short, well-filed nails are less likely to scratch open the skin.

‖‖➡ **If scratching is a problem, the person can wear clean white gloves.**

Wearing clean white gloves will help prevent scratching the skin with the nails. Gloves are especially helpful at night, when the person may not know he or she is scratching.

▟▶ **Change bed sheets daily.**

Dry skin flakes off and gathers on bed sheets, which can cause more itchiness and further dry out the skin. Changing the sheets frequently removes dry skin flakes and helps eliminate a buildup of bacteria. Fresh sheets bring a sense of comfort as well.

▟▶ **Encourage rest.**

Too much activity makes the skin sweat. Rest cools the skin down and decreases itchiness or skin irritation.

Take Steps to Manage Hand-Foot Syndrome

Hand-foot syndrome is linked to a number of cancer treatments, particularly some targeted therapies. Painful sensitivity in the hands and feet is the earliest symptom. The palms of the hands and soles of the feet may turn red and swell or blisters may develop. It is important to let the doctor know if the person is having any symptoms of hand-foot syndrome. Treating it early can help keep it from getting worse.

Encourage the person to take the following steps to manage hand-foot syndrome:

▟▶ **Wear shoes that fit well and aren't too tight.**

Thick soft socks may help if you have shoes that are big enough for the extra bulk.

▟▶ **Try gel shoe inserts if the soles of your feet are tender.**

▟▶ **Keep hands and feet moist by using mild skin creams.**

Try to pat the lotion into your skin—rubbing too vigorously can cause friction.

▟▶ **Avoid prolonged exposure to hot water on the hands and feet, such as with washing dishes or hot showers or baths.**

▟▶ **Avoid activities that put pressure on the hands and feet.**

For example, no running, aerobics, or jumping. Avoid massaging or rubbing your feet and hands. Also try not to use hand tools such as gardening tools or use knives to chop food—using these tools can put pressure on the hands.

▟▶ **Elevate your hands and feet when you're sitting or lying down.**

▟▶ **Apply ice packs wrapped in a towel to help cool burning hands and feet.**

▸ **Do not use harsh laundry detergents or cleaners, which can make the condition worse.**

▸ **Call the health care team if the person has any pain, swelling, redness, or blistering on the soles of the feet or palms of the hands.**

Help Conceal Dark Skin, Veins, or Discolored Fingernails

Skin pigment is affected by chemotherapy and often turns darker during treatment. If this side effect is bothersome to the person with cancer, suggest the following:

▸ **Wear long sleeves to hide dark veins.**
Long sleeves also provide some protection against bumping or bruising.

▸ **Apply a thin layer of makeup to the skin.**

▸ **Keep nails clean, short, and filed smooth.**
The person may want to wear nail polish.

Treat Acne

Changes in the pores and skin discharge can lead to blemishes that are both uncomfortable and unsightly. Encourage the person with cancer to take the following steps to prevent or treat acne:

▸ **Keep skin clean with mild soap and warm water.**
Harsh soaps inflame blemishes and strip the skin of important moisture.

▸ **Pat skin dry after cleansing.**
Gentle drying allows new skin to heal and doesn't irritate inflamed or swollen areas.

▸ **Avoid astringents.**
Although they dry out blemishes, astringents also dry the whole face and remove too much moisture. Keeping the skin clean is the best treatment.

Some targeted therapies can cause a rash that looks much like acne. Though the rash looks like acne, acne treatment medicines do not work on it—they can dry it out and make it worse. Some makeup brands, such as Dermablend, can cover the rash without making it worse.

Limit Sweating

If excessive sweating is a problem, encourage the person with cancer to do the following:

▸ **Dress in two light layers of clothing.**
Chemotherapy can cause excessive perspiration. The clothing layer closest to the body should be cotton to absorb moisture. The outer layer should be light to allow air to pass through.

▸ **Change damp or wet clothing or bed sheets as soon as possible.**
Damp or wet clothing or sheets can lead to chills and discomfort.

Limit Sun Exposure

Chemotherapy makes the skin tissue especially sensitive to the sun's rays, and sunburn can occur rapidly. Encourage the person undergoing chemotherapy to do the following:

▸ **Cover legs and arms when outside.**
Clothing stops the sun's rays from damaging the skin.

▸ **Wear lightweight fabrics.**
Lightweight fabrics allow more air to pass through to the skin and keep it dry.

▸ **Wear a wide-brimmed hat and sunglasses when outside.**

▸ **Use a sunscreen lotion with an SPF of 30 or higher that contains zinc oxide or titanium dioxide, applying it at least one to two hours before going out.**
Sunscreen prevents harmful rays from burning the skin. Remind the person to reapply sunblock at least every hour if he or she is sweating. Sunburn can occur in as little as fifteen minutes of direct sunlight. It is also important to apply sunscreen on overcast days, since ultraviolet rays can penetrate the clouds.

▸ **Cover newly exposed scalp.**
If the person has lost hair as a result of treatment, the exposed scalp will be very sensitive to the sun. The person should wear a head covering.

▸ **Stay in direct sun for only a short time.**

▸ **Stay out of the sun between 10:00 a.m. and 4:00 p.m.**
The sun is hottest and most dangerous during this six-hour period. People undergoing chemother-

apy, in particular, can be very sensitive to the sun's rays. Ask the doctor or nurse whether the person's chemotherapy regimen includes medicines that increase sensitivity to the sun.

Take Care of Skin During and After Radiation Therapy

Encourage the person undergoing radiation therapy to do the following:

⮕ Wash with lukewarm water and mild soap.

Wash the skin gently, and avoid very hot or cold water. Do not scrub the skin—scrubbing can cause skin irritation. Lukewarm water and gentle rinsing is best.

⮕ Keep the treatment area clean and dry.

A daily sponge bath or lukewarm shower is recommended. If any sweating occurs, clean and dry the skin gently.

⮕ Avoid using scented or medicated lotions, rubbing alcohol, scented creams or body oils, talcum powders, perfumes, and antiperspirants.

All of these products can irritate the skin. Many leave a coating on the skin that can interfere with radiation therapy or healing. Some special creams may be allowed by the radiation therapy department. Ask the staff for recommendations and instructions for use.

⮕ Do not use cornstarch to control perspiration.

Cornstarch will clump and cause a wet covering. Dusting with cornstarch or talcum powder is to be avoided. Report any problems with perspiration or dampness to clinic staff; they can suggest ways to deal with perspiration if it occurs near the radiation treatment area. Moisture is more likely to occur in skin folds, under the arms, and in the groin.

⮕ Avoid ice packs.

Ice irritates the skin. It constricts blood vessels and may inhibit healing.

⮕ Avoid hot water bottles and heating pads.

Heat can also irritate the skin.

⮕ Avoid direct sunlight to treated skin.

The layer of skin where radiation enters the body is very tender during and after radiation therapy. The ultraviolet rays of the sun can burn treated skin easily.

⫸ **Wear loose clothing.**

Tight clothing causes redness and irritation. Loose clothing lets the skin breathe and does not restrict movement.

⫸ **Avoid scratching treated skin.**

Scratching, rubbing, or scrubbing must be avoided. This friction can cause infection, irritation, or soreness. If itching is a problem, consult the doctor or nurse.

Possible Challenges

Consider the following situations that have been difficult for other caregivers:

"No one seems to know what to do about this itching. I guess we'll just have to live with it."
Itching is a difficult problem to resolve, but it can be improved. Try a combination of strategies to relieve constant itching. Keep experimenting and visit a dermatologist, if necessary.

"I'm afraid my skin will be fried by radiation therapy."
Radiation therapy does cause skin changes. The intention is not to "fry" the skin. Although it does get red and sensitive, the skin will heal. Be sure to ask for help, especially if the skin becomes sore or areas of moisture develop. Clinic staff will keep a close watch on the skin, and the radiation therapist may postpone treatment to give the skin a rest.

Carrying Out and Adjusting Your Plan

Think of other challenges that could interfere with carrying out your plan to manage skin problems. What additional roadblocks could get in the way of following the recommendations in this chapter? Will the person with cancer cooperate? Will other people help? How will you explain your needs to medical staff? Do you have the time and energy to carry out the plan? Develop plans for getting around these challenges by using the COPE ideas discussed in the introduction.

Check the skin regularly to see whether it has changed since radiation or chemotherapy began. Keep records of any skin problems the person is having and of what helps or makes them worse. These records will be helpful to health care professionals in diagnosing and treating any problems. If skin problems are getting worse, or if the person with cancer is becoming more uncomfortable or upset about these problems, review the section "What You Can Do." If you have done all you can, then ask the nurse or doctor for help. Discuss the results of your plan and what additional steps should be taken to manage the problem.

CHAPTER SIXTEEN

Loss of Appetite

Preparing food is often an important part of caregiving. It is a very personal way to show we care, and it is also important that the person with cancer eat as nutritiously as possible. How well a person eats is one indication of health. So it is natural for the caregiver to pay a lot of attention to how a person with cancer eats. It is important, however, not to focus too much on eating, especially if the person has little or no appetite. Too much pressure can make the person with cancer upset and can actually decrease his or her appetite. It is best to take a relaxed, positive attitude toward eating and appetite, even when it may be difficult. This chapter outlines things you can do to help increase the person's appetite and to increase the amount of nutritious food he or she eats.

People with cancer lose their appetites for many reasons. Cancer treatments and other medicines can decrease the desire for food, as can emotional distress or worry. Losing weight can upset the person with cancer and the family caregiver, especially if it is perceived as a sign the illness is getting worse. Rapid weight loss can often be slowed by taking steps to stop diarrhea, serving high-calorie and protein-rich foods, and taking medicines to increase appetite.

When to Get Professional Help

Call the doctor or nurse if any of the following conditions exist:

- ***The person has had very little to eat or drink for one day or more.*** You should ask the doctor or nurse when to report a poor appetite, but in general, you can use one day or more as a general guide. If nausea causes loss of appetite, read the chapter about nausea and vomiting for steps you can take to address that condition. If nausea lasts more than a few days and he or she is unable to eat very much, keep the doctor or nurse informed so the situation does not develop into an emergency.

- **Five pounds are lost in one week.** Ask the doctor or nurse when to call about weight loss, but in general, you can use five pounds in one week as a general guide. If the person with cancer is losing weight rapidly, inform a health care professional.
- **There is pain with chewing or swallowing.** Painful chewing or swallowing can interfere with normal eating and drinking. Pain can be caused by mouth sores or an infection on the tongue, gums, or throat. If there is a sudden change in appetite, ask the person if he or she is having trouble chewing, or swallowing.

Have the following information available before you call the doctor or nurse:
- When did the poor appetite problem start?
- How much weight has the person lost?
- Has this problem happened before? If so, what brought the appetite back or helped it improve?
- Does food taste different (for example, bitter or metallic)? If so, does this make foods less desirable?
- Which foods taste better or worse than they used to?
- Is the person's mouth dry or sore and is swallowing difficult?
- Does he or she have medicine to help with mouth problems? If so, what is the brand and dose?
- Does the person feel full or bloated soon after starting to eat?
- Is the person having nausea, vomiting, or problems with the bowels, such as constipation or diarrhea? If so, what medicines have been prescribed for these problems?
- When the appetite changed, was there a change in where or how food was eaten?
- Is the person's appetite better or worse at certain meals or at certain times of day?

What You Can Do

There are several ways you can help manage loss of appetite:
- **Help increase appetite.**
- **Encourage healthy eating.**
- **Minimize or eliminate bothersome tastes and smells.**
- **Prevent early feelings of fullness.**
- **Add protein and calories to the diet.**
- **Help with feedings and care of feeding tubes.**

Help Increase Appetite

There are several things you can do that will help stimulate a person's appetite.

▸ Encourage light exercise or walking before meals, in fresh air if possible.
Any increase in activity just before eating increases the appetite. Suggest a walk before meals, from five minutes up to thirty minutes.

▸ Eat meals with other people, whenever possible.
Avoid eating alone. Eating with someone else is distracting and can increase the amount a person eats by taking attention away from food. Sometimes meal habits change after a diagnosis of cancer because the family schedule is disrupted by trips to clinics for checkups and treatments. Returning to normal meal times and planning to have the family eat together can help increase the appetite.

▸ Eat meals in a pleasant, relaxed atmosphere, if possible.
A pleasant atmosphere can help to make food seem more appealing and take some of the attention away from food.

▸ Use small plates and serve small portions.
A small portion on a small plate can be arranged attractively and looks like a reasonable amount that can be finished.

▸ Keep food out of sight when not eating.
Keep food off countertops and put it in containers you can't see through. If the person with cancer doesn't see food all of the time, food may be more appealing at mealtimes.

▸ Drink lemonade or orange juice (if the mouth is not sore).
All juices contain acids that can stimulate appetites. Four ounces of juice before a meal may improve the appetite.

▸ Drink a small glass of wine, a beer, or a cocktail before lunch or dinner, if the doctor approves.
Alcohol stimulates the appetite. Alcohol should not be taken with certain medicines, however, and it should not be taken before chemotherapy treatments because it can cause nausea and even change the effect of the medicines. Ask the doctor about alcohol limits or about drinking any alcohol.

Encourage Healthy Eating

Good nutrition is important for people with cancer. Eating well helps them cope with the side effects of treatment. Healthy eating helps maintain strength, build immune system functioning, rebuild tissues, and speed healing. It is best if the person can eat a variety of types of foods.

➤ **Fruits and vegetables**

Fruits and vegetables provide important vitamins and minerals the body needs. Eating at least five servings of vegetables and fruits per day is recommended.

➤ **Protein**

Protein helps tissues heal and fight infection. Fish, chicken, meat, eggs, and cheese are good sources of protein. Eating three or more servings per day is recommended.

➤ **Grains**

Grains provide carbohydrates and B vitamins. Grains are a good source of energy. Examples of grains include bread, pasta, and cereals. Try to eat three to five servings of grains each day.

➤ **Dairy**

Dairy products are an important source of protein, calcium, and many vitamins. Examples include yogurt, ice cream, cheese, and other milk products. Eating two to three servings of dairy products each day is recommended.

Minimize or Eliminate Bothersome Tastes and Smells

Cancer treatments frequently change how foods taste, and smells (especially food smells) can become bothersome for the person. There are a number of things that can make food appealing again:

➤ **Use plastic instead of metal utensils.**

People undergoing chemotherapy may complain of a metallic taste in their mouth. Plastic utensils do not add to this bitter or metallic taste.

➤ **Try new spices and herbs, such as basil, curry, coriander, mint, oregano, or rosemary.**

Spices make our mouths water and change the taste of food. You may find a new spice or herb that makes the person hungry again.

⁞⁞⁞➡ **Add lemon juice or vinegars to vegetables and other foods.**

Sour flavors can make food taste better if treatment has made food lose its taste.

⁞⁞⁞➡ **Marinate meats in Italian salad dressing, mustard, sweet and sour sauce, soy sauce, or barbecue sauce.**

Sauces and marinades change the flavor of food and may make it more appealing. Strong flavors can also help to cut through "blah" tastes.

⁞⁞⁞➡ **Sprinkle more sugar and salt in food if these ingredients are not restricted.**

These seasonings can decrease the metallic and bitter tastes that people undergoing cancer treatment sometimes experience. Some people undergoing chemotherapy cannot tolerate sweet tastes, in which case they should use smaller amounts of sugar than before.

⁞⁞⁞➡ **Include carbohydrates and high-protein foods in the diet.**

High-protein foods include fish, chicken, meat, turkey, eggs, cheeses, milk, ice cream, tofu, nuts, peanut butter, yogurt, beans, and peas. Foods high in carbohydrates include bread, pasta, and potatoes. Try to get as much protein and as many carbohydrates as possible in each food item served. This strategy is called "powerpacking."

⁞⁞⁞➡ **Eat food cold.**

A cold temperature downplays the smell and taste of food. Aromas are blocked or linger for shorter times, and cold foods are not as flavorful, so odd tastes are covered up. The coolness also numbs the tongue to unpleasant tastes. Chicken salad, fruit salads, cold sandwiches, cereal, and yogurt are all good choices.

⁞⁞⁞➡ **Suck on hard, sugar-free sour or mint candy.**

These candies can mask strange tastes and may help if taken before a meal. These candies may also help the person cope with nausea and/or vomiting.

⁞⁞⁞➡ **Drink ginger ale or mint tea.**

Ginger ale and mint teas cover up metallic tastes and help make swallowing food easier.

⁞⁞⁞➡ **Avoid most red meats and serve chicken, fish, or pork.**

Changes in the taste buds may make red meat taste unpleasant. People undergoing chemotherapy often prefer chicken or fish.

➤ **If the person is sensitive to smells, prepare meals in a different room.**
Consider grilling outdoors or using a slow cooker on the back porch or in the garage to keep the aroma of food from permeating the inside of the home. Suggest that the person go to another room or to the opposite side of the house while food is being prepared. Remove any food covers to release food aromas before entering the area where the person will eat.

➤ **Sip broths or soups from insulated mugs with lids to block smells.**
Canned nutritional supplements can be put into cups with lids and drunk through a straw to minimize smells.

Prevent Early Feelings of Fullness

Poor appetite can be caused by an early feeling of fullness. Sometimes, medicines cause gas and the person can feel bloated after eating just a little bit. Several things can be done to help:

➤ **Exercise between meals.**
Any exercise gets the intestinal tract moving and shakes up pockets of gas. Even stretching and bending at the waist when standing up from a chair or couch helps relieve gas and move stomach contents downward.

➤ **Walk around or sit up for a while after meals, but avoid strenuous exercise immediately after eating.**
Walking or sitting up helps to empty the stomach and break up any gas, which can add to a sense of fullness and discomfort.

➤ **Drink beverages between meals instead of with meals.**
Liquids at mealtime can make the stomach feel full. Drinking less while eating allows more room for food.

➤ **Eat small amounts of food six to eight times a day.**
Small, frequent meals or snacks prevent an early sense of fullness, and more food can be eaten over the course of the day.

➤ **Avoid carbonation and certain vegetables.**
Cut back on fatty foods and such gas-producing foods and beverages as beans, cucumbers, green peppers, onions, broccoli, Brussels sprouts, corn, cauliflower, sauerkraut, turnips, cabbage, milk, rutabagas, or carbonated beverages. Some vegetables are digested slowly or create stomach and intestinal gas, which causes a feeling of fullness. Avoid carbonated sodas or waters, which can

make the stomach feel full when it isn't. Remove the carbonation by opening cans and bottles early, letting the fizz evaporate, and allowing the sodas to go flat. Avoid chewing gum, as air can be swallowed during chewing, which can lead to gas.

⟫ **Use over-the-counter medicines to help break up gas.**
Many products containing herbs or medicines that break up gas are available without a prescription. One particular ingredient found in some products, simethicone, is helpful in attacking gas and breaking up air trapped in the intestines. Check with the doctor and nurse before buying these over-the-counter medicines because they should not be used with some other medicines.

Add Proteins and Calories to the Diet

Rapid weight loss can often be slowed by adding calories and proteins to food. Encourage the person with cancer to do the following:

⟫ **Eat small, frequent snacks (six to eight per day) even if the person is not hungry, and encourage eating as much as is wanted.**
Smaller meals and snacks may result in more food consumption than restricting intake to three large meals.

⟫ **Encourage the person to choose snacks that are high in protein and calories.**
Examples include peanut butter, nuts or seeds, cottage cheese, canned nutritional supplements, or Instant Breakfast–type drinks.

⟫ **Add butter or margarine to vegetables, soups, pasta, cooked cereal, and rice.**
These fats add calories and improve the taste of many foods.

⟫ **Add sugar, syrup, honey, and jelly to vegetables, meats, cereals, waffles, and rolls.**
Sweet sauces add calories and can make dry foods easier to swallow.

⟫ **Use sour cream, cream cheese, ricotta cheese, or yogurt on baked potatoes, vegetables, and crackers.**
Creams are fattening, nutritious, and easy to swallow.

⟫ **Add whipped cream to hot chocolate, ice cream, pies, puddings, gelatin, and other desserts.**
Whipped cream is loaded with calories and has a pleasant taste. Add sugar to whipped cream to further boost calorie intake.

▸ **Add powdered coffee creamers or powdered milk to gravy, sauces, soups, and hot cereals.**

These products are good sources of calcium and increase the number of calories in food without adding bulk.

▸ **Use milk, soy milk, or plain yogurt instead of water to dilute condensed soups or cooked cereals.**

If a recipe calls for water, use these milk or soy products instead. This step will add calories and important nutrients and vitamins.

▸ **Use mayonnaise instead of salad dressing, and use half-and-half instead of milk in recipes.**

Mayonnaise and half-and-half have more fat and calories than salad dressing and milk. Avoid skim milk, if possible.

▸ **Add ice cream, tofu, ricotta cheese, or yogurt to milk drinks.**

These products increase the fat and calorie content in milk drinks and feel good on sore throats. Mix them well in a blender.

▸ **Add one cup of nonfat dry milk to one quart of whole milk for drinking and cooking.**

You can more than double the protein and calorie content of whole milk if you add powdered dry milk to it.

▸ **Use half-and-half or evaporated milk instead of water in recipes.**

Half-and-half and evaporated milk will add fat, protein, and calories. They also provide vital minerals and nutrients.

▸ **Spread peanut butter on crackers or bread, or use it on waffles, apple wedges, or celery sticks.**

Peanut butter is an excellent source of protein and calories.

▸ **Eat crushed granola, nuts, seeds, or wheat germ in shakes or on desserts.**

Nuts also are a great snack between meals.

⫸ **Drink nutritional supplements or your own milk shakes between meals or with snacks.**

Nutritional supplements, available as canned liquids or powders, are loaded with nutrients and can be purchased in most drug stores or grocery stores. Ask the nurse or pharmacist for specific product information. Drinking Instant Breakfast mixes is another way to get extra calories.

⫸ **Avoid diets designed to purge the gastrointestinal system.**

Certain diets are designed to purge or empty the intestinal tract. Unfortunately, these diets also remove essential vitamins, minerals, and fluids from the body.

⫸ **Ask the nurse or doctor about taking a vitamin supplement and iron.**

Vitamin supplements can help replace vitamins that are lost because of a suppressed appetite and reduced food intake. The doctor or nurse may suggest a daily multivitamin or iron pills as supplements to the diet.

Help with Feedings and Care of Feeding Tubes

If the person with cancer cannot swallow food, gastrointestinal (GI) tubes are sometimes used to transfer food to the stomach. GI tubes may be used temporarily, such as after surgery, or they can also be permanent. GI tubes are inserted into a hole that goes directly into the intestinal tract. A few times a day the tube is unclamped and connected to a bag holding a thick nutritious fluid that drips into the tube.

If nutrition support is necessary, a home health care nurse will instruct you in how to administer the feeding and how to care for the skin around the GI tube. You can ask for a home visit from a nurse to help you solve problems with this kind of feeding. For more information on nutrition support, visit the American Cancer Society Web site at **cancer.org**.

Possible Challenges

Consider the following situations that have been difficult for other caregivers:

"He says he's just not interested in food. He's not hungry at all."

Lack of interest in food cannot be changed easily. Try offering small snacks or meals in the company of people he or she enjoys. Try the other recommendations in this chapter. As difficult as it may be, do not focus too much on eating. Constantly talking about eating may turn off the person's appetite.

"Why bother with adding calories to food? The treatments make her so nauseated that she won't eat anyway."

Inform the doctor if nausea or vomiting is affecting the person's appetite. Some types of treatment may not cause the same upsetting side effects as others. New medicines to prevent nausea are also very effective. Adding extra calories to food helps prevent anemia and increases energy. It also helps keep weight on. All of these benefits help the person with cancer better handle treatments and feel better.

Carrying Out and Adjusting Your Plan

What additional challenges could interfere with your plan to manage appetite problems? What additional roadblocks could get in the way of following the recommendations in this chapter? Will the person with cancer be willing to try new foods? Are other people available to help with meal preparation? How will you explain your needs to a registered dietitian or other health care professional? Do you have the time and energy to carry out the plan? Develop plans for getting around these challenges by using the COPE ideas discussed in the introduction.

Keep track of the person's weight and the amount of food he or she eats. If problems occur, refer to the section "When to Get Professional Help." If you are not satisfied with the person's progress, talk about your concerns with the doctor or nurse. They may refer you to a registered dietitian who can help determine whether the person's diet is adequate and offer ideas to improve nutrition. The doctor may also prescribe an appetite stimulant or make other suggestions to help address this problem.

CHAPTER SEVENTEEN

Bleeding

Read this chapter in advance so that you are prepared if bleeding or bruising happens to the person with cancer. Sometimes you will need to act quickly to get medical attention. Sometimes you will have to deal with the bleeding yourself until you can get medical advice or help. There are also steps you can take to reduce the likelihood of bleeding or bruising. People undergoing certain kinds of chemotherapy are at higher risk for unusual bleeding, such as after shaving or brushing their teeth. Chemotherapy affects the bone marrow's ability to make platelets, which help the blood clot. Chemotherapy can cause the number of platelets to drop. Sometimes the doctor will prescribe medicines that increase the growth of platelets.

When a person receives chemotherapy, ask whether it will affect bleeding. If it does, ask the doctor when to get professional help if bleeding occurs, how to spot bleeding in its early stages, how to control bleeding, and how to help prevent it.

When to Get Professional Help

Call the doctor or nurse if any of the following conditions exist:

- *Any unusual or sudden bleeding lasting more than ten minutes, such as nosebleeds or bleeding gums.* Throughout the body, the blood flow system branches out into tiny capillaries. Most bleeding that we can see comes from these small blood vessels. The nose and mouth have many capillaries near the skin's surface. These places can easily break open and bleed.
- *Vomiting of blood or material that looks like coffee grounds.* In rare cases, bright red blood can be vomited. Blood in vomit, however, is more likely to be very dark in color and look like coffee grounds. This blood has been collecting in the stomach or abdomen and is likely caused by a bleeding ulcer or sore.

- **Blood in the urine.** Look for red, pink, or dark urine. Urine is usually light yellow. It is a darker yellow when the urine is more concentrated, for example, when a person is not drinking much fluid. Pink or red urine indicates a problem with bleeding. A change from yellow to dark urine should also be reported, although it may not be caused by blood.

- **Blood in the stool.** Look for red, dark red, or black stools. Bright red blood around a stool means blood vessels close to the rectum are open and bleeding. Hemorrhoids can cause these vessels to bleed. Dark black or tar-colored stools indicate a bleeding problem higher in the intestinal tract since the blood is older and darker by the time it comes out in the stool.

- **Tiny red spots on the skin (or in the mouth) or bruising, either of which appear quickly and without any apparent cause.** Tiny capillaries or blood vessels can open up in areas where they are closest to the skin's surface. When they bleed underneath the skin, they leave dots or spots that are red or purple.

- **Cough, sputum, or phlegm with blood.** Very small amounts of blood or streaks of blood may appear when the person with cancer coughs up phlegm (a thick, wet discharge produced in the respiratory system). If streaks of blood appear more than once or if the phlegm is quite bloody, report it to the doctor.

Have the following information available when you call the doctor or nurse:
- When did this bleeding start?
- How long did it last?
- How much blood was there?
- Has the person coughed up blood?
- For women, is there vaginal bleeding? How heavy is the flow?
- Is there bleeding anywhere else? If yes, where?
- What medicines were taken recently? At what dosage?
  - Aspirin
  - Ibuprofen, Motrin, Advil
  - Alka-Seltzer
  - Iron
  - Suppositories
  - Prednisone, Decadron
  - Nasal sprays
  - Sinus medicines
  - Arthritis medicines
  - Herbal medicines or supplements
  - Other medicines (explain what they are)

- Is the person receiving radiation therapy? If yes, where on the body and how recently?
- Has the person received chemotherapy recently? If yes, what type of chemotherapy and when was it received?
- Did the person with cancer have problems in the past with stomach ulcers or other bleeding problems?
- When were the last blood counts done, and what were the platelet levels?

What You Can Do

You can manage bleeding problems by following these guidelines:

- **Control bleeding when it occurs.**
- **Prevent bleeding.**

Control Bleeding When It Occurs

When bleeding starts, it often flows from tiny capillaries near the skin's surface, such as from the nose or gums. These capillaries open easily, but they also close easily. Try the following methods to stop the bleeding:

➧ **Apply pressure to the area of bleeding.**

Pressing on the skin gives the blood in the capillaries more time to clot. Using a clean, dry washcloth, apply pressure to the skin around the bleeding site for about four minutes. Do not look to see if the bleeding has stopped until four minutes have passed. You can also use an elastic bandage or gauze and firmly tape it around the wound, depending on where the bleeding occurs.

➧ Treat nosebleeds as described.

- *Sit upright and tilt head forward slightly.*
  Do not lie down or tilt your head backward because this causes blood to drip into the throat. Try not to swallow the blood during a nosebleed since swallowed blood can cause nausea and vomiting.

- *Pinch the nose closed and place ice on the bridge of the nose.*
  Pinch the nose closed with the thumb and forefinger for five to ten minutes. Put ice wrapped in a soft cloth over the bridge of the nose while you are pinching the nostrils closed. Do not check to see whether the bleeding has stopped or look at the nosebleed until at least five minutes have passed. In addition, ice on the back of the neck may help the person feel better.

Prevent Bleeding

The following actions can be taken to help prevent bleeding if chemotherapy has caused platelet counts to be low. These methods are not meant to be used regularly. Check with the doctor or nurse if you have questions.

▪▪▪➤ **Learn about blood counts.**

Ask the staff to explain platelet counts, what makes them go up and down, and what happens to a person with cancer as platelet counts rise and fall so that you will know when the person is at higher risk for bleeding problems. When platelets are low, the person will bleed more easily and will need to take special precautions, such as not playing contact sports or using softer toothbrushes until the platelet count is stable and normal again.

▪▪▪➤ **Do not use ibuprofen or ibuprofen products unless they are approved by the doctor.**

Ibuprofen-containing medicines include Motrin and Advil. Other nonsteroidal anti-inflammatory medicines (NSAIDs) you may want to avoid include naproxen (Naprosyn, Anaprox, Aleve), indomethacin (Indocin), sulindac (Clinoril), piroxicam (Feldene), or tolmetin (Tolectin). These medicines prevent the blood from clotting in the normal amount of time. Avoid giving these medicines when platelet counts are low.

▪▪▪➤ **Do not use aspirin or products containing aspirin (also called acetylsalicylic acid, ASA, or salicylate), unless they are approved by your doctor.**

These products include Alka-Seltzer, Percodan, Anacin, Ecotrin, Ascriptin, Excedrin, Fiorinol, Vanquish, and other drugs. Read the fine print on the label of any analgesic or pain relief pill. The label may list aspirin or acetylsalicylic acid as one of the ingredients, meaning the pill has aspirin in it. Aspirin makes a person bleed more easily, especially when platelet counts are low. Check with the pharmacist if you are not sure about a specific product.

▪▪▪➤ **If you need to take an over-the-counter analgesic, take aspirin-free products, such as acetaminophen (Tylenol, Datril Extra-Strength), and aspirin-free Anacin.**

Taking aspirin products can make bleeding happen more easily.

▪▪▪➤ **Do not floss teeth.**

Flossing can cut the gums, and bleeding may be hard to stop.

▪▪▪➤ **Use a soft toothbrush or Toothettes.**

Gums bleed easily when irritated or scraped. A soft toothbrush treats the gums much more gently, making them less likely to bleed. Toothettes are individually wrapped disposable oral sponges on sticks that may be substituted for a toothbrush when mouth tissues are sensitive.

⮞ Rinse and brush teeth after eating.

Rinsing helps remove leftover food, which can build up, start an abscess or sore, and make the gums bleed. Avoid mouthwashes that contain alcohol if the mouth is sore because they can burn the mouth. See page 149 for recipes for homemade mouthwash.

⮞ If the mouth is sore, eat soft, bland foods, such as soup, puréed meats, mashed potatoes, custards, gelatin, or puddings.

Soft foods are the least likely to cut or scrape the mouth. Bland, nonspicy foods are also less likely to cause bleeding; spicy foods can irritate the gums and lining of the mouth or cause pain and bleeding if the person has open sores or cuts. Avoid foods that are high in temperature, which can burn the skin of the mouth. When the platelet count is low, the skin can bleed when it is burned.

⮞ Use petroleum jelly or lip balm to keep the lips moist and to prevent cracking.

⮞ Remember to blow the nose gently and avoid nasal sprays.

There are many tiny blood vessels in and near the nose that can open up if the nose is blown too forcefully. Nasal sprays can cause nosebleeds if they are overused or are too strong.

⮞ Shave only with an electric razor.

Women can use hair removal products, such as Nair.

⮞ Avoid situations of potential harm and injury.

When the platelet count is low, it is important to use caution to prevent injury. For example, limit the use of sharp objects, such as razors, knives, scissors, or tools. Take a car or bus rather than ride a bicycle or motorcycle. Avoid contact sports. Ask others to do heavy lifting and strenuous activities. It is easy for small blood vessels to be damaged by bumps or falls.

⮞ Take steps to avoid constipation.

Straining to move the bowels can cause bleeding, especially around the rectum. See the chapter on constipation for ways to avoid constipation.

⮞ Pad the top of the hands with gauze if bumping them is likely to happen.

If the person bumps his or her hands frequently and bruising occurs, consider taping small pieces of gauze onto the tops of the hands as protection. Padding reduces the chance of bruising a vein and opening it up to bleed.

▐▶ **Do not use rectal thermometers, suppositories, or enemas or have rectal intercourse.**
Anything put into the rectum can tear its delicate tissues, and bleeding can start easily.

▐▶ **Do not use vaginal douches.**
Inserting items such as hard plastic douche applicators irritates sore skin in or around the vagina and can lead to bleeding.

▐▶ **Keep open cuts or scrapes clean to avoid infection.**

Possible Challenges

Consider the following situation that has been difficult for another caregiver:

"I need to take aspirin for my arthritis."
Many arthritis medicines put the person with cancer at risk for bleeding, but they can help control pain. If there is a history of bleeding problems, the person's risk of bleeding is greater. If pain control is important, this need may override the risk. This decision should be made only after consulting with the doctor. Ask about ways to control arthritis pain that do not increase the risk of bleeding.

Carrying Out and Adjusting Your Plan

Think of other challenges that could interfere with your plan to control or prevent bleeding. What additional roadblocks could get in the way of following the recommendations in this chapter? Will the person with cancer avoid potential harmful situations and prevent injury? Will other people help with heavy lifting and strenuous activities? How will you explain your needs to medical staff? Do you have the time and energy to carry out the plan? Develop plans for getting around these challenges by using the COPE ideas discussed in the introduction.

Keep track of the person's blood counts and chemotherapy dates to know when the risk for bleeding is higher. If problems with bleeding get worse, first ask yourself if you are doing everything possible to protect the skin from bruises, bumps, or cuts and to encourage good oral hygiene. Review the section "When to Get Professional Help." If you call the doctor or nurse, report the facts about the bleeding and what steps you have taken to manage this problem.

CHAPTER EIGHTEEN

Tiredness and Fatigue

Fatigue and feeling tired all the time are very common problems among people undergoing cancer treatment. People with cancer often say they feel more tired than they have ever felt in their lives. Fatigue caused by cancer is different from the tiredness that comes with everyday life. Cancer-related fatigue can appear suddenly and can be overwhelming. It is not relieved by rest, and it can sometimes last for months after treatment has ended.

There are some things you can do to reduce this feeling, but you can also help the person with cancer make the best use of the energy he or she has. You need to work together as a team to achieve this goal. Cancer fatigue is real and should not be ignored. It can be caused by a number of different factors, and it's not always possible to know exactly what the cause is. It may be caused by the disease itself or by the treatments. It may be caused by anemia, in which fewer red blood cells circulate and less oxygen is delivered to the body's tissues. Fatigue may be caused by malnutrition (inadequate intake of nutrients) or a temporary increase in waste products as cancer cells are destroyed by cancer treatments.

Sometimes, people feel tired after each course of cancer treatment. They complain of not having enough energy or not feeling like they can keep up with everyday activities. Fatigue may also happen because normal rest and sleep habits are disrupted or because the person with cancer is in pain or feels depressed.

Try not to push the person with cancer to do more than what he or she feels is reasonable. Let him or her decide how much to do. If other symptoms occur with increased fatigue, then it's important to talk with the doctor or nurse.

Recent research suggests regular exercise may help to reduce fatigue. While more research is needed to be certain, some studies have shown that people with cancer who participate in regular exercise programs have better physical performance and less fatigue than those who do not. Exercise strengthens muscles and adds flexibility. It may also help combat depression. However, people with cancer should talk with their doctors or nurses before starting an exercise program.

Exercise should not cause muscle strain or add to fatigue. Doctors and nurses who are familiar with the person's physical condition can judge whether exercise would be helpful and, if so, how much.

When to Get Professional Help

Tiredness or fatigue by itself is not an emergency; however, some symptoms can be serious if they occur in combination with tiredness. When these symptoms occur with fatigue, get **immediate help**. Call the doctor or nurse right away if any of the following conditions exist along with fatigue:

- *Severe or frequent dizziness.* Dizziness can happen when walking, getting out of bed, or moving from a sitting to a standing position. Dizziness can also occur without moving or changing one's position. Dizziness can happen to anyone occasionally. If it is severe and frequent, get medical help. Severe dizziness can be caused by a drop in blood pressure, not eating or drinking enough, or other physical problems.

- *Falling followed by an injury, bleeding, mental confusion, or unconsciousness.* Report all bad falls so the doctor or nurse can judge what caused the fall, whether bones were broken, and what follow-up is needed. Sometimes equipment may be recommended to prevent future falls. The doctor may refer the person to a physical therapist or occupational therapist for evaluation. See page 200 for information on what to do if a person falls.

- *Inability to wake up.* Call right away if you cannot wake the person or if his or her level of consciousness or alertness changes suddenly and unexpectedly. You will probably have to take the person to a medical facility for tests to determine the cause of this problem.

- *Feeling out of breath.* Breathlessness usually happens because the body is not getting the right amount of oxygen. This symptom can be caused by a problem with the lungs and respiratory system or by a low level of red blood cells.

- *Feeling as if the heart is racing with little activity.*

Other problems that might appear with fatigue that should be reported during **regular office or clinic hours** include the following:

- *Ringing in the ears.* This problem could be caused by a reaction to medicines, a change in blood flow to the brain, or other physical problems. Medical tests are usually required to determine its cause.

- *Pounding in the head.* This symptom could signal a problem with blood flow or blood pressure. Medical tests are usually required to determine its cause.

- **Staying in bed for days.** This behavior can be a sign of depression if it continues for days without other symptoms. See the chapter on depression if this behavior occurs.

Have the following information available when you call the doctor or nurse:
- How clear are the person's thoughts compared with before the symptoms began?
- Has confusion appeared or increased since fatigue began?
- Is the person with cancer feeling depressed or down?
- Has any new medicine been started, such as pain medicine or sleep medicine?

What You Can Do

You can manage fatigue by following these guidelines:
- **Help the person conserve energy.**
- **Promote sleep and rest.**

Help the Person Conserve Energy

Help the person conserve energy as much as possible.

Plan the day's activities so that being with people or traveling happens when he or she feels most refreshed and awake.
Allow time for rest between events.

Rest between bathing, dressing, and walking.

Engage in activities only for short periods.
Break activities into parts that can be done for a short time. Encourage the person to rest ahead of time.

Agree on what's most important.
Discuss which activities are most important or bring the most enjoyment. Start with the most necessary and enjoyable activities, and don't be disappointed if everything on the list doesn't get done. Be realistic in the goals you set.

Get up or move slowly to avoid dizziness.
Fatigue can cause dizziness. When the person is getting up from lying down, encourage him or her to sit on the edge of the bed and dangle the feet and legs for at least four minutes before standing up.

▐▶ **Plan regular exercise to reduce fatigue.**

Plan to do something every day, even if that only means getting dressed or walking out to sit on the porch. Short walks are also helpful. Ask the doctor or nurse about a moderate exercise plan.

▐▶ **Serve a balanced diet with adequate protein.**

Serve from the four food groups (dairy products; vegetables and fruits; breads, cereals, rice, and pasta; and proteins, such as meat, chicken, fish, or eggs). The most important nutrient is carbohydrates, which provide the most energy. Examples of foods high in carbohydrates are pasta, potatoes, bread, fruit, and energy bars.

▐▶ **Ask relatives and neighbors to bring food, or call a community meals program to deliver meals.**

Special menus are often available for people following low-sodium or diabetic diets.

▐▶ **Serve snacks as well as regular meals.**

Eating between meals is a good way to increase the amount of food eaten, which will help to give the person more energy.

Promote Sleep and Rest

Encourage the person to do some or all of the following:

▐▶ **Keep as active as possible during the day so that normal tiredness sets in at night.**

If the person remains active throughout the day, it will be easier to sleep at night.

▐▶ **Adopt an exercise plan that is approved by the doctor.**

Regular exercise can have a positive impact on better sleeping habits as well as reducing stress, anxiety, and depression. Ask the doctor or nurse for recommendations for a program that would be suitable for the person's condition.

▐▶ **Maintain regular patterns of rest and sleep as much as possible.**

Set regular times to nap and sleep, so the body comes to expect a routine. Routine habits help sleep.

▐▶ **Read the chapter on anxiety if nervousness or anxiety interrupts rest or sleep.**

Anxiety can make it difficult for the person to relax. Chapter 7 offers some good ideas on handling anxiety, including relaxation exercises. Talking with and being around other people can also help.

⟩ **Rest when tired—go to bed earlier, sleep later, and take naps during the day.**

If naps are a habit, taking longer ones allows more rest and helps to reduce fatigue. For some people, however, very long naps in the daytime can prevent sleep at night, so try to find a balance. Ask visitors to plan visits around sleeping and napping times.

⟩ **Play relaxing music before sleep.**

If certain sounds helped the person to relax and feel sleepy before the illness, make them part of the sleep routine now. Music or the sound of the television or of someone reading can be very soothing.

⟩ **Use a relaxation exercise before bedtime.**

See page 76 for a simple, effective relaxation exercise. Many relaxation exercises are also available as audio recordings and are available for purchase on the Internet or in stores.

⟩ **Drink warm milk at bedtime.**

Warm milk can be conducive to sleep.

⟩ **Take a warm bath or have a back rub at bedtime.**

These can be relaxing and can help the person feel more ready to sleep.

⟩ **Ask the doctor about sleeping pills.**

If the person tried the other things on this list and is still having trouble sleeping, ask the doctor if sleeping medicine would help. Do not give sleeping medicine without checking with the doctor first. These medicines can cause problems when combined with other medicines. Be sure the doctor is aware of all other medicines being taken when you ask about sleeping pills.

Possible Challenges

Consider the following situations that have been difficult for other caregivers:

"The fatigue comes with the treatments. There's nothing we can do to help it."

Cancer treatment often causes fatigue, but the person can control how that fatigue affects his or her life. The doctor also may be able to prescribe medicines to prevent anemia, which can cause or contribute to fatigue.

"There are so many things to worry about. No wonder I can't sleep."

Sleep often helps reduce anxiety because feeling tired can worsen anxious, jumpy feelings. Try to help the person make changes to promote better rest. Set up a regular bedtime routine, and encourage activities that reduce stress at bedtime, including taking a warm bath, reading, or spending time on a hobby.

Carrying Out and Adjusting Your Plan

Think of other challenges that could interfere with carrying out your plan to manage tiredness and fatigue. What additional roadblocks could get in the way of following the recommendations in this chapter? Will the person with cancer cooperate? Will other people help? How will you explain your needs to other people? Do you have the time and energy to carry out the plan? Develop plans for getting around these challenges by using the COPE ideas discussed in the introduction.

Keep track of how much of the day the person with cancer spends in bed. Check on whether current patterns of sleep and rest are similar to patterns before the illness.

If your plan doesn't seem to be working, you may be expecting change too fast. It usually takes time to work out ways to live with tiredness. Try to set reasonable, realistic goals for what you can accomplish. If tiredness is increasing and is of major concern to the person with cancer, ask the doctor or nurse for help. Tell the health care professionals what steps you have taken and discuss what additional steps could be taken to address the problem.

CHAPTER NINETEEN

Sleep Problems

People of all ages can have insomnia (trouble falling asleep or staying asleep). Stress, worry, changes in schedule or diet, or side effects of medicines or treatments are possible causes of insomnia. As people age, they generally spend less time in the deepest stages of sleep. After age forty, sleep becomes lighter, and it is easier to wake up. Sleep is considered a problem only when the person is not satisfied with his or her sleep, when the person feels drowsy the following day, or when the sleep problem suggests a serious underlying illness.

Sometimes, making a few simple lifestyle changes, such as getting more exercise during the day, is all that is necessary for a person to begin sleeping soundly. At other times, a problem such as stress, hormonal changes, poor nutrition, or drinking alcoholic beverages may cause insomnia. The most common reason for a sudden change in sleep patterns is stress or nervousness. Depression can keep people up and can wake them up at early hours.

Dementia frequently alters sleep patterns. A person with dementia may sleep during the daytime and then stay awake and even wander at night. Diuretics, antidepressants, anti-anxiety medicines, pain medicines, and drugs for Parkinson's disease also can affect sleep patterns.

Sometimes, people demonstrate odd behaviors while sleeping, which may be noticed only by a spouse or companion. Behaviors such as arm or leg movement, kicking, loud snoring, or choking sounds are signs of possible sleep disorders. These behaviors should be brought to the doctor's attention. One disorder to be concerned about is sleep apnea, a sleeping condition in which people briefly stop breathing. This condition causes them to wake up many times during the night. Sleep apnea can cause fatigue the next day and is associated with high blood pressure, heart disease, and heart failure.

When To Get Professional Help

Sleep emergencies are not common. However, call the doctor or nurse **immediately** or go to the emergency room if the following symptom occurs.

A sudden change in mood at night or bedtime. If the person for whom you are caring wakes suddenly during the night and acts agitated or confused, it is important to call a doctor right away. This change could be a sign of a serious medical illness or a side effect of a prescription drug.

Call the doctor **during office hours** to discuss the following problems:

- *Sleep is not satisfying.* Ask the person with cancer to explain what is not satisfying about sleep.
- *Sleep or fatigue cuts into daytime activities.* Falling asleep during quiet time, such as when watching TV, is normal, but falling asleep in the middle of a conversation is not. Excessive daytime sleepiness is abnormal. Falling asleep while driving, of course, is not only abnormal but also dangerous.
- *Strange behaviors occur during sleep.* Loud snoring, choking sounds, short periods when breathing stops, gasping, and wild leg and arm movements during sleep could all be signs of sleep apnea or other sleep disorders.

Have the following information available when you call the doctor or nurse:

- How long has sleeping been a problem?
- What other medical conditions does the person have?
- What medicines does he or she take? (Include prescription and nonprescription drugs.)
- Could stress be affecting sleep?
- Is he or she feeling sad, depressed, or anxious?
- Is snoring a problem? If yes, do you notice daytime drowsiness, choking, and/or gasping sounds during sleep?
- Are there complaints of indigestion, chest pain, or shortness of breath when the person wakes up during the night?
- Does the person consume or use alcohol, caffeine, or nicotine?

What You Can Do

You can manage sleep problems by taking the following steps:

- **Maintain a regular sleeping and waking schedule.**
- **Make the bedroom conducive to sleep.**
- **Pay attention to how diet and medications affect sleep.**
- **Encourage habits that can aid in sleep.**
- **Keep a sleep diary.**

Maintain a Regular Sleeping and Waking Schedule

A regular schedule can help prevent sleep problems.

➡ Encourage a set routine for going to bed and waking up.

As much as possible, the person should get up and go to bed at the same time every day. It is also important, however, that the person go to bed when he or she is sleepy. There is no need to lie in bed awake worrying about not sleeping.

➡ Develop a bedtime routine.

Activities like washing one's face, brushing teeth, or other nightly routines before bed help a person relax and prepare for bed.

➡ Get out of bed if not asleep in thirty minutes (if possible).

Getting out of bed and going into another room for a short period can help people who are having trouble sleeping. Listening to music or doing some light reading often helps feelings of tiredness to return. It is important to avoid bright light during these periods.

Make the Bedroom Conducive to Sleep

Follow these steps to make the bedroom conducive to sleep.

➡ Make the bedroom safe and comfortable.

Have a night-light in case the person wakes up confused or agitated. If the person wanders at night, be sure to secure doors and windows. Sometimes the noise of a fan running or a white noise machine helps people sleep.

➡ Use the bed only for sleeping.

Don't sit or lie in bed to eat, read, or watch TV. When the bedroom is used just for sleeping, it becomes associated with sleep, and that association can help the person with cancer feel sleepy when in the bedroom.

Pay Attention to How Diet and Medications Affect Sleep

Some medicines or substances in the diet could affect sleep.

➡ Check all medicines to see whether they could affect sleep.

Ask the doctor whether any medicines could be disrupting sleep. Some medicines, such as steroids, can prevent sleep. The doctor will want to know that sleep is a problem and will work with you to promote better sleep.

⟫ **Use sleep medicines with caution.**

Most prescribed sleep medicines are meant to be taken for no longer than two or three weeks. After three weeks, they lose effectiveness and can cause drowsiness during the day. Over-the-counter sleeping pills can cause dry mouth, constipation, urinary problems, and confusion.

⟫ **Limit or cut out alcohol, caffeine, and nicotine.**

These substances can interfere with one's ability to fall asleep and stay asleep, as well as disturbing the quality of the person's sleep.

Encourage Habits that Can Aid in Sleep

The following recommendations may improve the quality of sleep:

⟫ **Limit napping.**

Naps of up to one hour are often helpful, and naps taken in the middle of the day (at noon) are the most effective; however, napping for more than an hour can make it more difficult to sleep at night.

⟫ **Exercise.**

Exercise is a good remedy for poor sleep. A brisk walk in the afternoon is best. Exercising just before going to bed can cause difficulty in getting to sleep. If the person's ability to exercise is limited, then still encourage some walking and moving around.

Keep a Sleep Diary

Keeping a sleep diary should make clear when and how much sleep is being lost and how much sleep is gained during naps. Keep the following notes in a sleep diary:

- time the person woke up and went to bed
- how long it took to fall asleep
- the number of times awake during the night and the duration of the waking periods
- what woke the person during the night
- any strange behavior during sleep, such as choking or gasping sounds, stopped breathing, or leg movements
- characteristics of naps—when they were taken and how long each lasted
- alcohol, caffeine, or sleeping pill intake

A two-week sleep diary can help the doctor understand the problem and determine what treatments would be beneficial. Sometimes, a sleep diary can be reassuring because it shows that the person's sleep is better than previously thought.

Possible Challenges

Consider the following situations that have been difficult for other caregivers:

"If he stops taking sleeping pills, he won't be able to sleep."
Long-term use of sleeping pills may be contributing to or even causing problems with sleep.

"Sleeping problems are normal for older people."
Not true. Although there are some changes in sleep patterns as people get older, most sleeping problems can be solved or improved.

"She always takes a nap before supper."
The nap may be the reason for being unable to sleep at night. If the nap is a needed rest period, then it is okay. If napping is because of boredom, it may lead to less sleep at night.

Carrying Out and Adjusting Your Plan

Think of other challenges that could interfere with your plan to manage sleep problems. What other roadblocks could get in the way of following the recommendations in this chapter? Will the person resist changes to the sleeping routine? Will other people help keep a sleep diary? How will you explain your needs to medical staff? Do you have the time and energy to carry out this plan? You need to make plans for solving these problems. Develop plans for getting around these challenges by using the COPE problem-solving ideas discussed in the introduction.

Progress may be slow, especially at first. If you are setting up new routines to promote sleep, it usually takes time for people to get used to new routines and for the routines to be effective. Be on the lookout for sleep problems related to medical conditions or disorders, such as sleep apnea, which require medical treatment. Set realistic goals. A person is unlikely to suddenly begin sleeping eight hours at night if he or she has slept only four to five hours a night for years.

Be sure you have tried all of the suggestions in the section "What You Can Do." Be realistic about how quickly you can expect change. Brainstorm ideas of your own. You may find the best approach through trying different methods of problem solving. If problems with sleep are increasing and are of major concern to the person with cancer or are causing loss of sleep for you or other family members, ask the doctor and nurse for help. Discuss the results of your plan and what additional steps should be taken to manage the problem.

CHAPTER TWENTY

Hair Loss

Hair loss can be very upsetting to people undergoing cancer treatment. It is a highly visible reminder of the person's illness, both to him or her and to the outside world. As a caregiver, you can help by encouraging the person with cancer to prepare for hair loss before it happens. Knowing what to expect and being prepared for what happens can greatly reduce the stress and social isolation that can occur with hair loss.

Some chemotherapy treatments can cause partial or complete hair loss. This loss may start as early as seven to fourteen days after treatment begins, and hair may not grow back until some time after chemotherapy has ended. It may start to regrow during treatment. Radiation to the head can sometimes cause permanent hair loss. Other areas of the body can be affected as well. Depending on the type of chemotherapy or where the radiation is directed, eyelashes, eyebrows, and hair in the pubic area, on the arms, in the underarms, and on the chest and legs can be lost.

When hair does grow back, it may be different in texture. New hair may be a different color because of a temporary absence of pigment in the hair shaft. If hair was brown before treatment, it might grow back a lighter color. Changes in color and texture are usually not permanent.

Ask the doctor, nurse, or technician the following questions to learn more about the possibility of hair loss:

- Which treatments may cause hair loss?
- When will the hair loss start?
- Will it fall out suddenly or slowly?
- How much of the hair will be lost?
- When will it grow back?

When to Get Professional Help

Call the doctor or nurse if the hair loss is unexpected. You can also talk to a social worker or other mental health professional if the person with cancer feels extremely distressed about the hair loss or is having difficulty adjusting.

What You Can Do

You can manage hair loss by following these guidelines:

- **Care for the hair and scalp when the hair is falling out.**
- **Care for the exposed scalp.**
- **Help the person investigate wigs or head coverings.**
- **Take care of hair as it grows back.**

Care for the Hair and Scalp When the Hair Is Falling Out

Encourage the person with cancer to do the following:

➤ **Consider a shorter hairstyle before treatments begin.**

Time can help the person adjust to a new look.

➤ **Gently brush and wash away hair that is falling out.**

➤ **Gently clean hair and scalp with a mild shampoo twice a week.**

Use gentle shampoos for dry or damaged hair. Also massage the scalp to remove flaking dry skin.

➤ **Gently wash loose hair from other parts of the body using a mild soap.**

➤ **Use a satin pillow or hairnet while sleeping.**

A satin pillow prevents tangling, and hair sheds more evenly when held in a net.

➤ **Consider cutting or shaving the last few remaining hairs.**

When almost all hair is gone, the last strands can tickle or irritate the scalp, leading to scratching.

Care for the Exposed Scalp

During the time that the person is without hair, he or she should always do the following:

➤ **Protect the head and newly exposed skin from the sun with a hat and sunblock with SPF 15 or higher.**

The sun's rays can dry the scalp and burn it more readily than usual.

➠ **Wear a hat or a head scarf to retain heat in cold weather.**
Because heat is lost through the head, wearing a hat or scarf retains body heat. It also protects the scalp from drying out in cold, harsh weather.

➠ **Wear sunglasses to protect the eyelashes.**
Even eyelashes are sensitive to chemotherapy and can be easily broken. Protection from the sun and cold weather is recommended.

Help the Person Investigate Wigs or Head Coverings

Encourage the person to do the following:

➠ **Talk with other people who have lost their hair because of cancer treatments.**
People cope differently with this problem. Some accept baldness and do not cover their heads except in cold weather. Others feel wigs, turbans, or scarves are important and helpful. Getting ideas from people who have had the same problem can help the person judge what might be best for him or her.

➠ **If the person is interested in a wig, take steps before all the hair is lost.**
Ask a hairstylist about buying a wig, or call a wig shop and speak with the staff there. You can also call **800-227-2345** for help with finding a wig. Hairstylists can call a wig supplier and order catalogs. They can describe the different kinds of wigs to the person with cancer and order the wig. The wig can be matched to the person's hair color and texture. If you plan to buy a wig, be prepared to pay $50 or more. Synthetic wigs will be less expensive, whereas a wig made from human hair can cost several hundred dollars or more. Many people prefer to have their hairstylist order and style a wig specifically for them.

➠ **Find out whether the person's health insurance covers any costs of wigs.**
The health insurance company may provide partial or full payments for wigs if a doctor orders the wig.

➠ **Practice wearing the wig or other head covering at home.**
The person will be more comfortable in public after wearing the wig or other head covering at home and becoming used to it.

➠ **Try turbans, scarves, hats, and caps.**
Many stores sell attractive terry cloth or cotton turbans. Some hospital gift shops also carry these items. Head coverings protect against drafts, enhance appearance, and retain body heat.

LOOK GOOD...FEEL BETTER

Look Good...Feel Better is a free, nonmedical, brand-neutral, national public service program designed to help people going through cancer treatment look good, improve their self-esteem, and manage their treatment and recovery with confidence. Participants learn makeup and skincare tips and learn about hair care, hair loss, wigs, and head coverings. To find a program in your area, ask at your hospital or treatment center or visit **lookgoodfeelbetter.org**.

Take Care of Hair As It Grows Back

As hair grows back, encourage the person with cancer to do the following:

➠ **Use a protein conditioner.**
Conditioners add body to fine or limp hair. It takes time for new hair shafts to become thick.

➠ **Avoid hair care products that contain bleach, peroxide, ammonia, alcohol, or lacquer.**
Avoid hair dyes and products with harsh chemicals.

➠ **Select hairstyling products such as mousses, sprays, or gels that have light or normal hold.**
These products can be shampooed out. Stronger products build up on hair shafts and can damage remaining hair or new hair.

➠ **Avoid heat, curling irons, hot rollers, or blow dryers as much as possible.**

➠ **Gently towel dry hair or use a blow dryer set at the lowest setting.**
Keep heat farther away from the scalp than usual because the skin is sensitive and may burn easily.

➠ **Avoid braids or ponytails, and use a wide-toothed comb.**
Pulling breaks very fragile hair. Comb it gently with a wide-toothed comb.

➠ **Postpone a perm on new hair.**
If the person would like to get a perm, he or she should wait until new hair has grown to at least

three inches long to get a very mild body wave that will last for a short time. Permanent waves cannot be tolerated by the scalp until at least nine months after chemotherapy.

➡ **Keep hair short and easy to style.**
New hair breaks easily. Long hair requires more curling, pinning, and combing than short hair. Shorter hairstyles are easier to maintain.

Possible Challenges

Consider the following situations that have been difficult for other people coping with hair loss:

"I can't afford a wig."
Some insurance companies will cover part or all of the cost of a wig because it is needed after a medical problem and is not for purely cosmetic reasons. To get insurance coverage, you might need a prescription, so check with your doctor and insurance company.

"People say that he'll just have to live with being bald or having patches of hair on his head."
Appearance can be very important to all of us, including the person with cancer. Losing one's hair can be quite upsetting. Helping a person look his or her best during a difficult time in life can boost his or her spirits and provide confidence.

Carrying Out and Adjusting Your Plan

Think of other challenges that could interfere with carrying out your plan to manage hair loss. What additional roadblocks could get in the way of following the recommendations in this chapter? How will you help the person cope with the stress of hair loss? Will the person with cancer prefer a wig or other head covering? How will you explain your needs to professionals assisting with wig selection? Do you have the time and energy to carry out the plan? Develop plans for getting around these challenges by using the COPE ideas discussed in the introduction.

If possible, decide in advance whether the person wants a wig or other head covering and, if so, what kind. If the person is interested in a wig, order it as soon as possible. If hair loss is getting worse and the person is having difficulty coping or adjusting to this change, ask your social worker or nurse for help. Discuss the results of your plan and what additional steps could be taken to address the problem.

CHAPTER TWENTY-ONE

Mobility Problems and Falls

People with cancer can experience a variety of physical problems at different times during the course of treatment and over the length of illness. Problems with mobility and balance can be particularly discouraging and potentially dangerous. Problems moving around, bathing, keeping balanced upright, or getting up from the bed or furniture because of fatigue or balance problems are very real concerns for many people during cancer treatment. A person who is weak or unsteady on his or her feet is at high risk for falling. Some of the most common situations in which falls occur are trying to get out of bed, falling off the toilet, slipping in the bathtub or shower, and tiring out while walking and falling.

Helping the person in the bathroom or when moving around the house can be a challenge to many caregivers. If you have a bad back or health problems that prohibit lifting or straining, helping the person with cancer may be especially difficult. There is equipment available to make walking, bathing, and moving from one place to another safer and easier for both of you. It is a matter of knowing what is available and learning how to use the necessary equipment to the best advantage.

When to Get Professional Help

Call the social worker or nurse if any of the following conditions exist:
- *You are not able to help the person move from one piece of furniture to another.*
- *You are not able to get the person from the house to the car.*
- *The person has fallen repeatedly or has been hurt in a fall.* (See page 200 for more information on what to do if the person falls.)
- *The person with cancer needs supplementary oxygen, and it is difficult for you to help him or her move around with the oxygen equipment.*
- *The person has new weakness or numbness.*

- ***The person has new dizziness, problems with balance, or disorientation.***

What You Can Do

You can manage mobility and balance problems by following these guidelines:

- **Assist the person in moving around.**
- **Take steps to ensure a safe home environment.**
- **Use equipment to make movement easier at home.**
- **Know what to do if the person falls.**

Assist the Person in Moving Around

Help the person move around to avoid falls.

➠ Ask the person to ask for help getting up or walking if he or she feels weak or off balance.

➠ When the person needs to get out of bed, have him or her sit on the side of the bed for four minutes.
This will help if the change in position causes dizziness or unsteadiness.

➠ If the person is feeling lightheaded, stay with him or her in the bathroom.

Take Steps to Ensure a Safe Home Environment

Some falls can be prevented by ensuring a safe home environment.

➠ Inspect the bathroom and stairs for safety.
Most accidents happen either in the bathroom or on stairs. Make sure objects on the floor are removed and railings are secure.

➠ Install handrails in the shower or tub.
Many people hang onto racks or shelves in the tub for steadiness. However, shelves or racks can weaken and be pulled down. Handrails can be placed over the sides of the tub or installed directly into the bathroom wall or the shower stall.

➠ Place nonslip appliqués on the tub floor.
Appliqués can be purchased at most pharmacies, supermarkets, or hardware stores and decrease the chance of slipping while showering or getting in and out of the tub.

▸ Remove or secure throw rugs and other objects that can cause the person to trip.
Loose rugs are easy to slip on, especially when they are on linoleum or wood floors. Walking paths should be clear of clothing, throw rugs, and other items that could cause tripping or slipping. Keep electrical cords off the floor and tape the edges of rugs to the floor.

▸ Use a stable shower chair in the bathtub.
Shower chairs make bathing or showering much safer. The larger the chair, the steadier it will be. Some shower chairs are even made to stretch over the side of the tub so a person can sit on a bench and slide over into the tub without as much lifting or shifting of body weight.

▸ Install a showerhead with a flexible hose that can be held in the hand and directed to specific areas of the body.
A flexible showerhead that can be lowered to the person is safer and more efficient than trying to use a stationary showerhead.

▸ Use wheelchairs or commodes with lift-off arms and lift-off footrests.
Chairs with lift-off arms and footrests can be positioned alongside the bed or couch. The person can lift the arm of the wheelchair or commode and easily slide over to the new seat.

▸ Raise beds, toilets, chairs, and couches to make it easier to move on and off of them.
Getting out of a bed that's at a low height can be difficult. Raising the bed on wooden blocks can make for a safer and easier transfer. Toilets also are often too low, and a raised toilet seat can be purchased to elevate the seat anywhere from four to six inches. Chairs and couches can be dangerously low and lead to strains and even fractures when one is trying to rise out of them. Again, wooden blocks can be placed under furniture to raise it to safer heights.

▸ Try sliding boards between seats to help with awkward transfers.
Sliding boards are short pieces of wood that stretch between a wheelchair, for example, and a bed. The person does not have to stand to get from one place to another but scoots across the board to the new setting.

▸ Make sure the person wears shoes or nonskid slippers when walking.
Avoid slippery shoes or open-heeled slippers.

▸ Consider using the Lifeline service to get help from neighbors.
Subscribers to Lifeline wear a button on a cord around their neck or keep it near them so they

can signal a neighbor for help in an emergency. Most local community hospitals have this service. Look in the telephone book, on the Internet, or call the hospital and ask for the Lifeline telephone number and contact person. Someone will interview you over the telephone and explain the monthly rental service. Sometimes financial discounts are available. You will need to name three neighbors who will agree to keep a key to the home and respond to a call from a central operator if the button is pushed. This system is an alternative to calling 911 or the emergency response unit.

Use Equipment to Make Movement Easier at Home

Many types of equipment can be used at home to make moving around easier.

➡ Ask whether the hospital or home care agency has its own supply store.
Some hospitals and agencies have their own supply stores as well as personnel who will help customers learn about different options for home care.

➡ Call a local medical equipment store to find out what products they have to help with moving and walking.
Most medical supply stores can advise you over the telephone about equipment options for use at home. They may be able to help you determine which types of equipment would be covered by insurance and whether a doctor's prescription would be necessary.

➡ Consult a home care catalog for ideas.
Many pharmacies and some large retailers produce catalogs and Web sites that picture and describe a variety of home care equipment and devices.

➡ Ask service groups about donated equipment.
Different service groups collect and repair equipment such as wheelchairs and commodes. Ask your social worker or look on the Internet to find out whether there are groups in your community that could provide the equipment you need.

Know What to Do If the Person Falls

If the person falls, follow these guidelines:
- Leave the person where he or she has fallen until you can determine whether there are serious injuries.
- If the person is unconscious, bleeding, or has fluid draining from the mouth, ears, or nose, call the doctor or 911 right away.

American Cancer Society

- If the person is not breathing, call 911 unless the person is in hospice or has a durable power of attorney for health care that states his or her wish not to be revived.
- If the person is conscious, ask if he or she feels any pain.
- Check the person's head, arms, legs, and buttocks for cuts and bruises and to see if anything looks strange or misshapen (possibly because of a broken bone).
- Apply ice packs and pressure to any bleeding areas. Put ice in a plastic bag and wrap the bag in a towel.
- If you cannot move the person, make him or her as comfortable as possible until help arrives.
- If the person is not in pain, is not bleeding, and does not seem to have suffered any serious injuries, help him or her back to bed or to a chair. If possible, have two people move the person.

Possible Challenges

Consider the following situation that has been difficult for another caregiver:

"My father won't use the equipment I got to help him get around."

Discuss the problem together and what you can do to deal with it. If he does not agree there is a problem, explain your concerns about his safety. Ask him to use the equipment for your sake. If he cannot understand your point of view, get help from other people, such as other family members, friends, or health care professionals. If he does not want other people to see him using the equipment, put it away when there are guests. If he forgets to use the equipment, find ways to remind him—for example, putting up signs—or he can practice using the equipment until it becomes habit.

Carrying Out and Adjusting Your Plan

Think of other challenges that could interfere with carrying out your plan to manage mobility problems and falls. What additional roadblocks could get in the way of following the recommendations in this chapter? Will the person with cancer use the equipment? Will others help the person with cancer get around? How will you explain your needs to equipment suppliers? Do you have the time and energy to carry out the plan? Develop plans for getting around these challenges by using the COPE ideas discussed in the introduction.

Work with the person to develop plans to deal with problems moving around and prevent falls. Try simpler solutions first—things you can do together with what you have in your home. Talk with nurses, social workers, physical therapists, or occupational therapists, and ask for their suggestions. Look into borrowing equipment. If it can't be borrowed and it is going to be needed for only a short time, consider renting. Purchasing equipment can be cheaper if it is needed for a long time.

Keep track of the problems the person has walking and moving. For problems that happen only occasionally and are not dangerous, you may want to wait to see whether they become more frequent. If a problem is potentially dangerous and you are worried, develop a plan before the problem becomes serious.

If your plan does not seem to be working or the person's mobility problems are getting worse, review the section "When to Get Professional Help" in this chapter. If any of the conditions listed there exist, call the social worker or nurse immediately. If problems with moving around the house continue, ask the social worker or nurse for help. Discuss the results of your plan and what additional steps should be taken to solve the problem.

CHAPTER TWENTY-TWO

Veins and Vein Punctures

M any chemotherapy treatments are injected into veins, and veins are used to obtain samples for blood tests and other diagnostic tests. In this familiar procedure, known as venipuncture, a needle is inserted into a vein to withdraw blood or to give medicine or other fluids. The person with cancer may feel anxious about needles and vein punctures. Family caregivers can be helpful by encouraging the person, helping him or her relax before and during the vein puncture, and helping to prepare skin and veins for vein punctures, thereby limiting discomfort.

It is important to protect the veins of anyone undergoing cancer treatment. Treatment can cause veins to become sore or difficult to find or use. This chapter explains what you can do to minimize these problems, as well as some alternative ways to give or get blood or medicines that do not require repeated needle punctures. After treatments are over, most people's veins return to normal. In some cases, veins are damaged for a long time. Chemotherapy sometimes causes sclerosis of the veins, which means they harden and cannot be punctured again.

Vein punctures are, for the most part, unavoidable. As a caregiver, you can help prevent undue anxiety about this procedure and help the person with cancer protect his or her veins.

When to Get Professional Help

The following three symptoms indicate a serious skin or vein problem. Each needs to be evaluated and treated by a health care professional. Call the doctor or nurse if any of the following conditions exist:

- *Aching, tenderness, swelling, or redness (particularly a red streak) anywhere on the arm where the needle entered the skin.* The nurse will need to decide whether the person needs to come to the clinic to have the arm or vein inspected. These symptoms might mean the skin or vein is reacting to the drug. The staff can also tell you over the phone how to treat the problem, perhaps by putting an ice pack on the skin or using warm compresses.

- *Any drainage, pus, or blisters at the site where the needle punctured the skin.* Clear or yellow liquid coming from the needle insertion site could mean an infection.
- *Anxiety about needles is severe enough for the person to consider skipping treatments or procedures.* A few people become so anxious about having their blood drawn it stops them from going to a clinic appointment, visiting the laboratory, or having blood drawn. The health care team can help deal with this problem; address it early, before it interferes with treatment.

Have the following information available when you call the doctor or nurse:
- When did the skin or vein problem start?
- Where are the sore veins?
- When was the procedure that made the site sore?
  - If chemotherapy, what type was it?
- Is there a black or dark blue bruise or any red streaks?

What You Can Do

You can manage veins and vein punctures by following these guidelines:
- **Prepare for vein punctures.**
- **Limit discomfort and anxiety during vein punctures.**
- **Learn about alternatives to repeated vein punctures.**
- **Learn how to care for intravenous (IV) tubes and feeding tubes.**

Prepare for Vein Punctures

Encourage the person with cancer to follow these guidelines to prepare the skin and veins for punctures:

▶ **Stay warm just prior to vein punctures.**
Warmth makes the veins relax and fill with blood. Sometimes, chemotherapy nurses will wrap the arm in a warm, wet cloth a few minutes before an injection. This step helps the veins be seen more easily.

▶ **Eat well the day before treatment.**
Food and fluids help maintain good blood flow through the veins. On the day of treatment, the person with cancer should eat and drink normally in the morning unless he or she is scheduled

for tests that require fasting (going without food for a period of time).

⟱ Drink two to three quarts (eight to twelve glasses) of liquid every day, if possible.
Fluids dilate, or inflate, the veins. Blood flows better, and the veins are more likely to stick up and be found easily. Encourage the person with cancer to drink as much as possible, unless fluids are restricted for other reasons, such as heart disease.

⟱ Take a walk while waiting for chemotherapy or a blood draw.
Walking helps increase good blood flow and keeps the veins pumped up.

⟱ Exercise the hands and arms at home.
Exercising at home can help veins inflate. Encourage the person to squeeze a rubber ball or lift small weights, such as cans of soup. This exercise can be done while talking with family or friends or watching television.

⟱ Use moisturizing lotions.
Apply lotion, cream, or ointment to the skin from fingertips to elbows. Lotion keeps the skin moisturized, which prevents dryness, cracking, and thickening of the skin. When the skin is dry, it is harder, and needle punctures are more painful. The best time to apply moisturizers is after the skin has been wet—after bathing, showering, swimming, or doing dishes. Pat the skin almost dry and then apply the lotion. Use lotion as often as possible—at least four times each day.

Limit Discomfort and Anxiety during Vein Punctures

Needles and vein punctures make many people anxious. Encourage the person with cancer to do the following to reduce or minimize anxiety:

⟱ Take anti-nausea medicines, which also promote relaxation.
Check with the doctor or nurse about taking anti-nausea medicines before chemotherapy treatments. Many of these medicines also decrease anxiety.

⟱ Talk about pleasant experiences while waiting.
Have the person talk or think about pleasant experiences while waiting for a treatment or blood draw.

⟱ Do activities to take the mind off treatment.
Reading an interesting magazine or talking with another person in the waiting room about something pleasant can help. Bring a portable music player to listen to music or relaxation recordings.

▥➡ **Look away from the arm during the vein puncture.**

Many laboratory workers and nurses distract the person undergoing vein puncture by talking with him or her. Suggest the person also look somewhere else in the room during the procedure.

▥➡ **Talk to the doctor about the anxiety.**

The doctor may prescribe a medicine to help the person relax or may recommend a mental health professional to help with these feelings.

▥➡ **Practice deep breathing and relaxation techniques, and use these skills when receiving intravenous (IV) treatments or undergoing vein punctures.**

Relaxation is a skill and improves with practice. Practicing at home will make it easier to use that skill to relax in medical settings.

▥➡ **Ask about the use of products that numb the skin, such as topical anesthetics, if vein punctures are very painful.**

The doctor may be able to prescribe a product such as EMLA cream, which numbs the skin and can be used prior to procedures involving vein punctures.

Learn about Alternatives to Repeated Vein Punctures with Needles

If vein punctures are so troubling or difficult that going to the laboratory, undergoing treatments, or having transfusions is a continuing problem, or if the person is facing a large number of these procedures, there are other ways to give and get blood and medicines.

▥➡ **Ask about alternatives to vein punctures.**

Finger sticks" for some blood draws.

Sometimes a "finger stick"—a pin prick on the finger that gives only a drop or two of blood—is all that is needed for certain tests, such as a complete blood count or platelet count. Ask the nurse or laboratory technician if this method is an option for some tests.

IV catheters that connect to large veins.

These catheters are small, flexible, sterile tubes that can be put into large veins. They are the same size as most IV lines. The tubes can stay in for months and are taped to the chest or arm. These catheters, sometimes called "Broviac catheters," "Hickman catheters," or "PICC lines," are used to draw blood and to inject chemotherapy medicines. Some people choose to have these catheters inserted to avoid repeated vein punctures in the arms and hands.

Permanent ports or access devices placed under the skin.

Another way to get medicines into the body without sticking a vein every time is through a permanent port site. Ports are small metal discs, usually about one inch in diameter, that are placed under the skin, most often on the chest. A small IV line extends from the port into a large vein. If you press lightly on the skin, you can feel the port, but it is barely visible from the outside.

If an IV catheter or a permanent port is being considered, review the following questions to help determine which method is a better choice:

- ***How often does the catheter or port need to be flushed to stay open, and who will handle this task?*** Ports need to be flushed only once every four weeks if no medicines have been given and no blood has been drawn. The person can visit a doctor's office or clinic and have this task done. A nurse can also flush the port at the person's home if the person is unable to travel. Some patients or caregivers learn to do this task themselves, but it takes good control of the fingers and good vision to flush a port alone. IV catheters in the chest must be flushed every day to keep them open and available for future use. The dressing around them needs to be changed three times per week. Caregivers and family members can learn to do this task at home.

- ***How much can a person move and exercise with catheters and ports?*** Ports do not prevent athletic exercise. Because the port is under the skin, the person can swim, play sports, and do any athletic activity he or she wants. Catheters hang outside of the body, so swimming and some athletic sports are not advised because the catheter might be pulled out during the activity.

- ***Will treatments be better with catheters or with ports?*** Some medical centers require a catheter be used with certain medicines. People with leukemia, for example, need to have a catheter inserted to receive large amounts of IV fluids and medicines. Ask which method the medical center prefers to use, and use the one it recommends.

Learn How to Care for Intravenous (IV) Tubes and Feeding Tubes

If the person is receiving medication or nutrition support by IV or feeding tubes when at home, you will have to learn how to manage their care. Nurses can show you how to care for the skin around the tubes and how to mix and give medicines or food through the tubes. If you have problems, you can ask for a nurse to visit the home to help you solve problems.

Possible Challenges

Consider the following situations that have been difficult for other caregivers:

"The staff didn't say anything about ports or catheters, so I assumed that they couldn't be used."
The staff may not know how upsetting vein punctures are to the person with cancer, so they may not think it is a problem. If it takes three or more attempts to access a vein in the arms, ask about the availability and advisability of using a port or catheter.

"I've had trouble with needles all my life, so nothing can be done."
Health care staff who give cancer treatments are usually very experienced doing venipuncture. They have had special training in how to do this procedure, and they understand how difficult vein punctures can be for some people. Therefore, you may find vein punctures in a cancer clinic are much less of a problem than you thought they might be.

Carrying Out and Adjusting Your Plan

Think of other challenges that could interfere with carrying out your plan to manage veins and vein punctures. What additional roadblocks could get in the way of following the recommendations in this chapter? Does the person have trouble with needles? Would a port or catheter be preferred over repeated vein punctures? Will other people provide helpful distractions during treatment? How will you explain your needs to medical staff? Do you have the time and energy to carry out the plan? Develop plans for getting around these challenges by using the COPE ideas discussed in the introduction.

Review the suggestions in this chapter regularly, and monitor the person's experiences with vein punctures. Are nurses and laboratory technicians able to find veins during blood draws and chemotherapy treatments? Is the person worried or upset about vein punctures? Have alternatives to needles been considered? If problems with veins are getting worse or the person is becoming more anxious, review the recommendations listed in this chapter. If you have done all you can, then ask the nurse or doctor about the different options for IV lines or ports on a short- or long-term basis.

CHAPTER TWENTY-THREE

Confusion and Seizures

Mental confusion during cancer treatment is not common. Mental confusion and communication problems can be caused by medicines, strokes, changes in body chemistry, or the presence of cancer in the brain. Lack of sleep can add to disorientation, as can new and unfamiliar surroundings.

If confusion does happen, it can be upsetting to both the person with cancer and caregivers. Confusion also can cause communication problems that are frustrating for everyone. Sometimes, this problem can lead the person with cancer to stop trying to communicate. Family caregivers may be tempted to give up on communication as well, but you should understand that steps can be taken to cope with these problems.

Although very rare, seizures can occur in people with cancer. If they do occur, they are likely related to some problem with the central nervous system. A seizure can be very frightening for both the caregiver and the person with cancer. Preparing for a seizure in advance is wise, especially if the treatment staff warns that a seizure may happen.

Confusion and seizures, if they do occur, may not be related to the cancer treatment, but they are important symptoms that need to be addressed, whatever the cause.

When to Get Professional Help

Call the doctor or nurse if any of the following conditions exist:

- **The person experiences a sudden change in the ability to speak after starting a new medicine.** This symptom should be reported to a doctor or nurse. The medicine may be the cause of the problem, and the doctor may need to adjust the doses and the medicines being taken.
- **Mental confusion increases or is new.**
- **The person demonstrates clouded thinking or disorientation.**

- **_The person's personality suddenly and dramatically changes._** The cause of this behavior may be a physical change in the brain, emotional problems such as depression, a medicine, or a stroke.
- **_The person's ability to manage routine tasks or care for him or herself suddenly changes._** If the person suddenly needs assistance with tasks that have typically been managed alone (such as dressing or washing), a doctor may need to determine whether there is a physical cause for this change.
- **_The person falls because of confusion._** Mental confusion increases the likelihood people will not know where they are. Climbing out of bed or getting up and walking can cause a fall. Speak to your health care team about whether a nurse or home health aide might be able to come to your house and help you make the rooms safer to navigate. If the person does fall, make him or her comfortable on the floor by using pillows and blankets and then call for help. See page 200 for more information on what to do if the person falls.
- **_Long pauses or slurred words begin to characterize speech._** Changes in the ability to speak can happen suddenly or develop over a short period, such as over the course of several days. Problems speaking can result from a stroke, in which the brain does not get enough blood or oxygen. Recognizing changes in speech may be difficult because the person may be sleeping more and talking less in general. Try to watch for any changes. If a person who typically uses complete sentences suddenly begins speaking in short words, using sentences that make no sense, or babbling, seek professional help. Other symptoms of a stroke are sudden numbness or weakness on one side of the face or body, sudden trouble seeing in one or both eyes, sudden trouble walking or dizziness, and sudden, severe headache with no known cause.

Have the following information available when you call the doctor or nurse:
- When did the confusion or word slurring start?
- Were any new medicines started? If so, which ones, when, and at what dosage?
- Has the person changed where he or she is living?
- Have other changes occurred in the person's setting? If so, what are they?

What You Can Do

You can manage confusion and seizures by following these guidelines:
- **Make it as easy as possible for the person to understand others.**
- **Help the person avoid becoming confused.**
- **Know what to do if a seizure occurs.**

Make It As Easy As Possible for the Person to Understand Others

Use these techniques to make communicating with the person easier.

▶ **Use simple words and short sentences.**

Short words and sentences are easier to understand. Ask questions one at a time, and wait for an answer. Try not to give complex choices or combine questions. For example, instead of asking, "Do you want to lie down now or have Fred visit?" you can just ask, "Do you want Fred to visit now?" Avoid treating an adult like a child or using baby talk.

▶ **Use a picture or the real thing to get your message across.**

If the person does not seem to understand a simple question, show something to help get the message across. For example, if you want to know if he or she would like something to drink, show a glass of liquid.

▶ **Minimize distracting noises in the room.**

If others are talking and a TV or radio is blaring, it will be hard for anyone to hear a conversation or question. Keep this in mind if the person is having difficulty understanding someone else's speech.

▶ **Explain to visitors or other caregivers how they can help the person with cancer hear and understand better.**

Explain that hearing or talking is a problem, and explain how you cope with confusion and improve communication.

▶ **Tell the person with cancer what you are going to do before you do it.**

Before you move the person or help him or her do something, explain what is going to happen. It can help a confused person to have some advance warning before such changes as getting out of bed or serving a meal. Try, however, not to treat the person like a child. Just use simple words and explain what is going to happen. For example, "I'm going to help you out of bed now."

▶ **Try not to argue.**

It is easy to lose patience with someone who is not mentally clear or keeps forgetting what you say. Arguing, however, can increase anxiety and actually make it harder for the person to understand what you are saying.

Help the Person Avoid Becoming Confused

Take these steps to help avoid confusion.

⟫ Try to keep the person awake during the day and asleep at night.
Many people who are very sick get night and day mixed up, and this mix-up can add to their confusion. Try to keep the person awake during the day, so he or she can sleep at night. This way, routines such as mealtime or bath time will not seem disorienting.

⟫ Use a night-light in the person's bedroom to help him or her see and recognize surroundings.
A person who is confused can sometimes wake up and not recognize his or her surroundings. A night-light gives just enough illumination to help the person see and get oriented.

⟫ Keep the person's surroundings as familiar as possible.
Unfamiliar people or surroundings may cause confusion. For example, if the person goes to a nursing home or a hospital, take along pictures, photographs, favorite pillows, or covers and use them in the new setting to retain some familiarity.

⟫ Keep a clock and a calendar within sight.
It is easy to lose track of the time of day and the day of the week. Clocks and calendars can help prevent confusion.

⟫ Continue giving medicines on a regular schedule.
If the person is experiencing any confusion, it can be difficult to keep track of multiple medicines. You may need to help monitor when the person takes required medicines.

⟫ Give any medications prescribed to prevent or reduce confusion.
Some medicines may be prescribed to reduce confusion. Steroids, such as prednisone, decrease swelling or inflammation in the brain. If confusion or problems with talking are caused by a cancer in the brain, it is important to keep giving medicines that keep any swelling from getting worse.

⟫ If the person has lost weight, ask whether medicine doses need to be adjusted.
The dose for a medicine may change depending on a person's weight. If the person is losing weight, the dose of some medicines may be too large, which could cause confusion. Perhaps dosage sizes could be lowered without losing their desired effects.

Know What to Do If a Seizure Occurs

Follow these steps if a seizure occurs.

⟶ Place a soft washcloth in the person's mouth.

The purpose of placing something in the mouth is to prevent the person from biting his or her tongue or lips during the seizure. However, do not try to force the mouth open if it is closed.

⟶ Do not put your hands in the person's mouth.

Do not try holding the person's tongue or mouth with your hands, which could result in your being bitten.

⟶ Clear the area of any hazardous items.

Remove any hard or sharp items from the area around the person.

⟶ Turn the person gently onto one side.

This will help keep the airway clear.

⟶ Put pillows on both sides of the body.

Pillows will help keep the person in place and, if he or she is in the bed, help prevent him or her from falling out.

⟶ Place something flat and soft under the person's head.

This could be a small pillow or a folded towel or shirt.

⟶ Pad any side rails on the bed with soft blankets.

Metal side rails on hospital beds can hurt and bruise the person if he or she bumps them. Padding the side rails is a good idea if you think seizures may occur.

⟶ Do not try to hold the person down or stop his or her movements.

⟶ Tell others how to handle seizures.

Keep a list near the person's bed of what to do if a seizure occurs. Keep a soft washcloth nearby. If volunteers or others who are not the usual caregiver stay with the person, give them these instructions.

Possible Challenges

Consider the following situations that have been difficult for other caregivers:

"Why bother to explain anything? He doesn't know where he is or who I am."
Confusion can come and go, so you will not always know whether the person is confused at that particular moment. Explain things, and talk with him as an adult even if you are not certain he understands you.

"Why talk about the past? She can't even remember where she is now."
Remembering the distant past might be easier for her than remembering what happened yesterday. In general, this is true for many older adults (those eighty-five years or older). Talking about the past can be pleasant and comforting as well, and it can bring tears as well as laughter. If other friends or family are present, they also will enjoy the stories and learn more about her.

"I feel so sad that he doesn't know who I am."
It is sad to feel that someone no longer remembers or knows you. This change can make you feel like you have lost someone. Maybe there were things you wanted to say or do together, and you now wonder whether it is worth it. Confusion can come and go. Say those things anyway, and hope your words are understood as coming from you.

Carrying Out and Adjusting Your Plan

Think of other challenges that could interfere with carrying out your plan to manage confusion and seizures. What additional roadblocks could get in the way of following the recommendations in this chapter? Will the person with cancer resist changes to the routine? Will other people know what to do in the event of a seizure? How will you explain your needs to medical professionals? Do you have the time and energy to carry out the plan? Develop plans for getting around these challenges by using the COPE ideas discussed in the introduction.

Be patient and creative. It will take time to discover the best ways to communicate with someone experiencing confusion. Be realistic in your expectations. Look for signs the person recognizes you and understands what you have said. Keep track of what causes any improvements. If communication and confusion remain problems, ask the doctor or nurse for further suggestions and guidance. They have experience communicating with people who are confused and will know what you can realistically hope to achieve.

Part IV

Living with Longer-Term Side Effects of Cancer Treatment

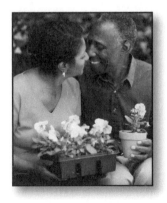

THIS SECTION PROVIDES INFORMATION ABOUT LIVING WITH SOME OF THE LONGER-LASTING EFFECTS OF CANCER TREATMENT. The chapters include lymphedema, ostomies and prostheses, and sexual conditions. Encourage the person with cancer to read this information, and then you can work together as a team.

Each chapter is organized under five major topics:

1. Understanding the condition
   - when the problem will likely occur
   - what kinds of things can be done to help
   - what goals to have when dealing with the condition

2. What you can do
   - what you can do to manage the problem at home
   - what you can do to help to prevent the problem

3. When to get professional help
   - when to call for help immediately
   - when to call during office hours
   - what information to have ready when you're calling

4. Possible challenges
   - recognizing problems
   - how to deal with problems you may have in carrying out your plans

6. Carrying out and adjusting the plan
   - how to monitor progress,
   - how quickly to expect change
   - what to do if the plan isn't working

The information in this section fits most situations, but your situation may be different. If the person's doctor or nurse provides different instructions, always follow the advice of your health care providers. For more information on coping with cancer and cancer treatment, contact your American Cancer Society at **800-227-2345** or visit the Web site at **cancer.org**.

CHAPTER TWENTY-FOUR

Lymphedema

Lymphedema is the swelling of any limb or limb part (such as the hand, wrist, arm, ankle, calf, or leg) due to insufficient drainage of the lymphatic system. It can happen if the person has had lymph nodes removed during surgery or if the person has undergone radiation treatment that has damaged or caused swelling in lymph nodes. Lymphedema is most common among women who have been treated for breast cancer. These women may experience swelling of the arm and/or hand on the side of the body where the breast cancer occurred. Lymphedema can also develop in men treated for prostate cancer and people treated for abdominal or pelvic tumors. These people may experience swollen ankles or legs as a result of lymphedema.

The onset of lymphedema is often subtle and unpredictable. There is no way of predicting who will or will not develop lymphedema. It can happen immediately after treatment or months or even years later. The potential for developing lymphedema continues throughout the person's lifetime, and lymphedema can have a profound effect on the person's quality of life. There is no cure for lymphedema, though it can be managed. With proper education and care, many people can avoid lymphedema or, if it develops, keep it under control.

This chapter will discuss what lymphedema is, the steps that can be taken to lower one's risk of developing lymphedema, the signs to look for, and how to manage lymphedema if it occurs.

What Is the Lymphatic System?

The lymphatic system is a network of thin vessels, lymph nodes (also called "lymph glands"), and lymph fluid. The lymphatic system helps fight infection by circulating and filtering lymph, a clear liquid that carries immune cells throughout the body. The lymph fluid is removed from and returned to the blood through the lymph vessels. When the lymphatic system is damaged, the lymph fluid does not drain properly and builds up in the limbs, making them swell.

Signs of Lymphedema

These are some of the signs of lymphedema:

- Swelling in an extremity
- Feelings of fullness or heaviness in the area
- Changes in skin texture or appearance (such as tightness, firmness, or redness)
- New aching or discomfort in the area
- Less movement or flexibility in nearby joints
- Trouble fitting the limb into clothing or the bra doesn't fit the same
- Ring, bracelet, or watch feels tight even though the person has not gained weight

Treatment of Lymphedema

Damage to the lymphatic system cannot be repaired. If lymphedema is diagnosed, the goal of treatment is to control swelling, keep it from getting worse, and decrease the risk of infection.

Mild swelling can sometimes be improved by keeping the swollen arm or leg elevated as much as possible. Prop the arm or leg on a pillow. This position will make it easier for fluid to drain from the swollen area.

Lymphedema can be treated by a physical therapist or health care professional who has gone through special training to deal with lymphedema. Treatment methods include the following:

- a compression sleeve that helps push fluids out of the swollen area
- manual lymphatic drainage (performed by a trained therapist), which involves gentle massage to direct and stimulate lymphatic drainage
- use of a sequential gradient pump, which reduces swelling by applying pressure to the limb in timed cycles

Most insurance companies will pay for lymphedema treatment, but some do not cover the cost of compression garments. Consult your insurance provider to find out what is covered.

When to Get Professional Help

Call the doctor or nurse during office hours if any of the following conditions occur with the person:

- ***Any swelling, tightness, redness, or signs of infection on the affected arm or leg.*** These signs could indicate infection on or under the skin. The limb with lymphedema can become infected more easily than other limbs, and it is important to report an infection in the early stages so it can be treated.
- ***Any injury to the arm or leg that is affected by lymphedema.*** Injuries include punctures from pointed objects, sunburns, or cuts and scratches from pets, sharp objects, or

knives. These injuries should be reported to a doctor or nurse who can decide whether an antibiotic is needed or tell you what to watch for signs of infection.

- **Pain or discomfort caused by swelling from lymphedema.** Pain or discomfort can be a sign of infection. If the swollen skin aches or is tender to the touch, there may be an infection. Pain may signal an infection before you can see swelling. Pain could also be caused by a backup of fluid in the limb or could be a sign of other problems that the doctor should investigate.
- **Temperature of 100.5°F or higher (when taken by mouth) that is not related to a cold or flu.** Fever can be a sign of infection.

Have the following information available when you call the doctor or nurse:

- What surgery or radiation treatments has the person with cancer had and where in the body?
- What things were done in the past to manage the lymphedema, and how successful were they?
- What has been done to control lymphedema during this episode, and what have been the results?
- If the problem is an injury, when did the injury occur, and what has been done?

What You Can Do

At this time, there are no studies showing that lymphedema can be prevented. Most experts, however, say that following some basic guidelines can lower the risk of lymphedema or delay its onset.

- **Avoid infections in the limb.**
- **Avoid burns.**
- **Avoid constriction.**
- **Avoid muscle strain.**
- **Avoid gaining weight.**
- **Take proper care of any cuts, scratches, or burns.**

Avoid Infections in the Limb

The body responds to infection by making extra fluid. Removal of or damage to lymph nodes makes it harder to move this extra fluid, and it can trigger lymphedema. Good hygiene and skin care can help to reduce the chance of infection and reduce the risk of lymphedema. Encourage the person to do the following to avoid infections:

▐▶ Do not allow blood draws, needle injections, or blood pressure cuffs on the limb where lymph nodes have been removed or radiation was given.
Punctures or pressure on the limb can cause swelling and infections. Tell technicians, nurses, and doctors that you are at risk for lymphedema so that they can avoid hurting the affected area.

▐▶ Keep the affected limb clean and dry.
Wash daily if the limb is sweaty or dirty. Dry the skin well after washing; damp skin lets bacteria grow. Keep feet clean and dry, and wear cotton socks.

▐▶ Use moisturizing lotion.
Overly dry skin gets infected more easily because bacteria can enter through cracks in the skin. Lotion helps keep the skin flexible and prevents cracking. For best absorption, apply when the skin is still slightly damp from bathing or washing hands.

▐▶ Avoid using sharp objects near the limb. Be very careful using needles, pins, and knives.
Use a thimble when sewing to avoid needle and pin pricks to your finger. Any cuts or abrasions will heal slowly, and infection is more likely to set in when the limb is affected by lymphedema.

▐▶ Use insect spray when outside.
Biting insects can pierce the skin, and the skin will heal slowly if affected by lymphedema. The bites can also cause infections. If you are stung by a bee on the affected limb, clean the area and put ice on it, raise the limb, and call the doctor or nurse if the sting shows any sign of infection.

▐▶ Clip and manicure nails carefully.
Avoid tearing or cutting cuticles, which could cause infection. Instead, use a lanolin-based cream to soften cuticles. Push your cuticles back with a cuticle stick rather than cutting them with scissors. Cut toenails straight across, and see a podiatrist as needed to prevent ingrown nails and infections.

▐▶ Use an electric shaver to shave near the affected limb.
An electric razor is less likely than razor blades to damage the skin. For example, women who have had a mastectomy should use an electric razor to shave under the arms.

▐▶ Wear gloves when gardening.
Unprotected hands are more likely to be cut or punctured by thorns, sharp leaves, or gardening tools.

▪▶ **Wear rubber gloves when working with household cleaners, detergents, and bleaches.**
Household cleansers are very drying and can damage and crack the skin. Loose-fitting gloves will protect the hands and will prevent skin damage from harsh chemicals.

Avoid Burns

Burns can also cause the body to make excess fluid, which can increase risk of lymphedema. Encourage the person to avoid burns by following these guidelines:

▪▶ **Wear protective clothing and sunscreen when in the sun.**
Avoid exposure to the sun between 10 a.m. and 4 p.m., when the sun is most likely to burn the skin. Use a sunscreen with SPF 30 or higher and zinc oxide or titanium oxide for activities in the sun, and apply sunscreen at least one to two hours before going out.

▪▶ **Keep bathwater and dishwater lukewarm.**
Hot water can scald the skin. Scalded skin cracks and peels and is likely to become infected in a limb with lymphedema. Avoid testing bathwater or dishwater with the affected limb.

▪▶ **Use oven mitts and potholders.**
Oven mitts and potholders protect the skin from burning and scalding.

▪▶ **Avoid high heat, such as from hot tubs or saunas.**
Heat can increase fluid buildup. Also avoid using heating pads on the affected areas.

Avoid Constriction

Constriction of the limb can increase the pressure in nearby blood vessels, which may lead to increased fluid and swelling. Lymphedema has also been linked with air travel, possibly because of low cabin pressure. Encourage the person to follow these guidelines to avoid constriction:

▪▶ **Wear loose jewelry, clothing, and gloves.**
Avoid anything that forms a snug band around the affected limb.

▪▶ **Do not use shoulder straps when carrying briefcases and purses.**

▪▶ **Wear a loose-fitting bra with padded straps that do not dig into the shoulder.**
People who have had mastectomies should wear lightweight prostheses.

⟫ **Do not have your blood pressure taken on the affected arm.**
If both arms are affected, blood pressure can be taken on the thigh.

⟫ **When traveling by air, wear a compression sleeve.**
A well-fitted compression sleeve may help prevent swelling by helping to squeeze the lymphatic fluid through the remaining vessels before it builds up. Careful fitting is required, however; a garment that is too tight near the top can actually reduce lymph flow. Ask the doctor or physical therapist about getting fitted for a sleeve to wear during air travel. There are also ways to safely raise the arm above heart level and exercise it during long flights.

Avoid Muscle Strain

⟫ **Use the affected arm or leg as normally as possible.**
If the arm or leg with lymphedema is not used, muscles will become weak, and weakening may increase the likelihood of bruising or damaging the limb. Regular exercise can help keep the muscles toned.

⟫ **Avoid heavy lifting.**
Heavy lifting will strain the limbs and pull muscles. Heavy packages or suitcases should be carried with the unaffected arm or side.

⟫ **Avoid scrubbing with the affected arm.**
Scrubbing, pushing, or pulling with the affected arm can make it swell more and can damage muscles.

Avoid Gaining Weight

Studies have linked weight gain after mastectomy to a higher risk of lymphedema. Extra fat requires more blood vessels, which creates more fluid and places a greater burden on the remaining lymph vessels.

Take Proper Care of Any Cuts, Scratches, or Burns

If the person does get a cut, scratch, or burn, proper care is very important. Wash the area with soap and water, and put an antibiotic cream or ointment on the area. Cover with clean, dry gauze or a bandage. For burns, apply a cold pack or cold water for fifteen minutes, then wash with soap and water and put on a clean, dry dressing.

Watch for signs of infection, such as redness, rash, swelling, tenderness, increased heat, pus, chills, or fever. Call the doctor right away if infection is suspected.

Possible Challenges

Consider the following situations that have been difficult for other caregivers:

"He forgets to do everything he needs to do to control his lymphedema."
Family members and friends can remind the person with lymphedema about what to do. Putting a list of recommendations someplace where it can be seen and noticed may help.

"She gets so upset by her lymphedema that she doesn't want to think about it—and so she doesn't do some things she should to control it."
Encourage the person to separate in her mind the things she needs to do to control the condition and the actual lymphedema. Encourage her to think of these activities as part of her normal routine. Also, she can enlist family and friends to offer reminders without mentioning lymphedema.

Carrying Out and Adjusting Your Plan

Think of other challenges that could interfere with carrying out your plan to help prevent or manage lymphedema. What additional roadblocks could get in the way of following the recommendations in this chapter? Will the person take steps to avoid injury and infection? Develop plans for getting around challenges by using the COPE ideas discussed in the introduction.

Controlling lymphedema takes time and patience. Look for small changes and improvements. Lymphedema problems will probably continue, but your goal is to help the person have an improved quality of life and for the episodes of swelling to be less severe.

If lymphedema problems continue or if they are happening more often, encourage the person to talk to the doctor and ask for a referral to a physical therapist. Be sure the person is following the recommendations provided by the doctor and physical therapist, as well as those listed in this chapter. If so, keep following them. Even if problems continue, you can prevent lymphedema from becoming worse.

CHAPTER TWENTY-FIVE

Ostomies and Prostheses

Ostomies and prostheses are two different ways to help people return to a normal life after having organs or body parts removed by surgery. An ostomy is a surgical opening in the body. Prostheses are man-made substitutes for body parts that have been removed. Both require learning to use the new body part, and both can require an adjustment in lifestyle.

An ostomy is a surgically created opening that leads to the urinary or gastrointestinal tract or into the trachea. The whole apparatus—from the skin to the internal organ—is called an ostomy. The "stoma" is the part of an ostomy that you see on the skin. Ostomies are created to remove fluid or feces from the body or to allow air into the lungs. These are the most common types of ostomies:

- **Tracheostomy:** A surgical opening in the neck to the trachea to create an airway
- **Colostomy:** A surgical opening from the large bowel or colon to the abdomen to allow fecal matter to pass to the outside of the body
- **Ileostomy:** An opening in the ileum (part of the small bowel) to the abdomen that allows small bowel contents to pass to the outside of the body
- **Urostomy:** An opening in the urinary system where urine can pass to the outside

Some other, less common types of ostomies include jejunostomy and gastrostomy. Some ostomies are temporary and are used to give the body time to heal. Once the body heals, the ostomy is closed and the body resumes its normal function. Other ostomies are permanent, such as when an organ must be removed. The person with cancer, along with the caregiver, must learn how to care for the stoma.

Prostheses replace body parts that have been removed. Examples include breast, testicular, and leg prostheses and penile implants. The original body parts are sometimes removed because they contain cancer that can spread.

When to Get Professional Help

Call the doctor or nurse during office hours if any of the following conditions exist:

- **The person with cancer is having difficulty caring for an ostomy or stoma.** Health care professionals, such as respiratory therapists and nurses, can teach the care of tracheal ostomies, and enterostomal therapists and other nurses can teach the care of urinary or colon ostomies. These professionals can visit the home if needed. Ask the doctor or nurse to arrange a teaching session.
- **The area around the stoma becomes red or swollen, is itchy, or develops bumps or a rash.** These symptoms could be caused by infection. They also could be caused by the pouch not fitting correctly, or they could be a skin reaction to the pouch or adhesive.
- **A prosthesis scrapes the skin or causes redness or pain.** This discomfort means the prosthesis is not fitted correctly and needs to be adjusted.
- **The person with cancer is confused about the type of prosthesis to purchase.** Talking with a doctor or nurse can help the person with cancer decide on a type of prosthesis that best meets his or her needs. The doctor may refer the person with cancer to a specialist and may also recommend local support groups where people with the same conditions help support each other.

What You Can Do

There are some things you can do at home to help the person with an ostomy or prosthesis:

- **Learn to care for the ostomy.**
- **Help the person with cancer make a decision about and/or select a prosthesis.**
- **Support the person in learning to cope with an ostomy or prosthesis.**
- **Support his or her decision.**

Learn to Care for the Ostomy

⟹ Tracheostomy

- **Assist with the care of a tracheal ostomy following a total laryngectomy.** Family caregivers should know how to care for a tracheal ostomy and be available to help the person when needed. Encourage the person to follow these guidelines to care for the tracheostomy:
  - Clean the tracheostomy tube at least once a day as instructed by the doctor.
  - Suction the tube as needed or as directed to clear mucus that can build up at the top of the windpipe.

- Gently clean the skin around the opening every day or as directed.
- Be careful to keep water out of the tracheostomy. When bathing, a waterproof child's bib with the plastic side facing outward can be used to keep water out and allow the person to breathe. The person should not swim.
- Keep the air in the home and bedroom moist by using a humidifier. Keeping the environment moist will help reduce problems with thick crusted mucus.
- Wash hands carefully before and after handling the tracheostomy to prevent infections.
- Encourage the person to wear a scarf or shirt that covers the opening that is made of thin fabric (such as cotton) to allow air to get through. This helps protect the stoma from dust and loose fibers.

Urostomy

- **_Be available to assist with the care of urinary diversions._**

Urinary diversions drain urine out of the body through a stoma on the skin. Drainage is collected in small plastic pouches that are worn at all times. Learn how to care for the ostomy and offer to help if the help is needed or wanted. Encourage the person to do the following to care for the urostomy:

- Every day, gently clean the skin around the stoma with warm water only. Gently pat dry or allow to air dry. Showers or baths can be taken with the pouch on or off. The skin must be thoroughly cleaned when the pouch is changed.
- Apply barriers, borders, or pastes to the skin around the stoma before putting on the pouch.
- Empty the pouch when it is one-third full.
- Change the pouch every three to five days.

Colostomy and ileostomy

- **_Assist with the care of colostomies._**

Colostomies and ileostomies are surgically created openings of the bowel. Many people wear a colostomy pouch over the stoma to collect the feces that empties into the pouch. Others learn to regulate bowel movements so a pouch does not need to be worn at all times. Caring for the skin around the stoma and getting the right kind of pouch can be challenges in the beginning. Sometimes the person with the colostomy is embarrassed to have help. If so, explain that you are available to help if it is needed or wanted. Encourage the person to follow these guidelines:

- Every day, gently clean the skin around the stoma with warm water only. Gently pat dry or allow to air dry. Showers or baths can be taken with the pouch on or off. The skin must be thoroughly cleaned when the pouch is changed.

- Apply barriers, borders, or pastes to the skin around the stoma before putting on the pouch.
- Empty the pouch when it is one-third full.
- Change the colostomy pouch before there is a leak—if possible, at least every three to four days and no more than once a day.
- Irrigate the stoma as directed.

Help the Person Decide About or Select a Prosthesis

There are many different types of prostheses. Some are external (worn outside the body), and others are implanted during surgery. The most common types are breast, testicular, and leg prostheses and penile implants.

➡ **Help with choosing a breast prosthesis, if appropriate.**

Breast prostheses can be internal (breast implants) or external.

External breast prostheses

External prostheses vary in type, weight, and color. Some replace an entire breast, while others are small and worn by women after a lumpectomy or a segmental mastectomy. There are also nipple prostheses for when the nipple cannot be saved during breast reconstruction. Choosing a breast prosthesis is an important personal decision. As a family caregiver, your support and encouragement can be very helpful—though it is important the woman make her own decision. One advantage of external prostheses is that they can be easily replaced if they are not satisfactory.

External prostheses are sold in surgical supply stores and lingerie shops. Call ahead to find out whether they carry the type of prostheses desired and whether they have a professional fitter. Sometimes a custom-fitted prosthesis is needed. Encourage the person with cancer to follow these guidelines:

- ***Compare types of external breast prostheses and prices.***
  Suppliers differ in the prices and the help they give. Shop around for the best fit and the right price. Using the telephone or Internet to do research will save time and trips.
- ***Wear a formfitting top when shopping for an external breast prosthesis.***
  A formfitting top will show the fit of a prosthesis, which should be natural in contour and shape. A snug top will also help the person with cancer see whether the prosthesis stays in place when she moves.

Breast implants

Breast implants are prostheses that are surgically inserted under the skin. They can be removed with surgery but generally are left in for life. Some women prefer a breast implant to an external breast prosthesis because the implant creates a more natural appearance without clothes. A breast implant is also more convenient since there is no need to put on and take off the prosthesis every day. The decision to have breast implants is a very personal one. Since breast implants can be inserted at any time, there is no rush to make a decision. However, there are more options available if implants are discussed at the time of diagnosis and treatment. She may want to experiment with an external breast prosthesis before deciding whether she wants an implant. For more about breast implants and breast reconstruction, visit **cancer.org** or call **800-227-2345**.

Support His or Her Decision

The issue of prostheses can be a personal and delicate issue. For men, the decision to have or not have a testicular or penile implant is both personal and sensitive. Not all men feel they need or want an implant; however, for some, having the implant is very important. Likewise, some women choose not to use a prosthesis or get an implant after having a breast procedure such as a mastectomy. There is no right or wrong choice, but it can be a deeply personal and important issue. As a caregiver, you can help by supporting whatever decision he or she makes. Most types of implants can be done at any time, so there is no rush in making a decision.

Support the Person in Learning to Cope with an Ostomy or Prosthesis

Learning to live with an ostomy or prosthesis can be an adjustment, and your support is important.

⏵ **Talk about the prosthesis.**

Sometimes, people are hesitant to talk about getting a prosthesis. They may feel embarrassed or not want to upset others. You can help by expressing your willingness to talk about it—when he or she is ready and willing. You can say you understand why the person feels hesitant but also explain that talking openly can help him or her think through the options and make a better decision.

⏵ **Offer support while the person learns to use a new leg or arm prosthesis.**

Temporary leg or arm prostheses are usually fitted immediately after surgery that removes a limb. Permanent prostheses are fitted later after the wound has healed. In either case, it takes a while for a person to get used to using the new artificial limb. During this time, emotional support from family caregivers is very helpful. You may also be able to help put on the prosthesis when he or she is learning to use it.

⫸ **Encourage the person with cancer to join a local ostomy club.**

In these groups, people with ostomies help each other by giving support and sharing experiences. Ostomy clubs can also be found by looking online, calling your American Cancer Society at **800-227-2345**, or contacting the social services department of your local hospital. Another group that can help you find a local club is the United Ostomy Associations of America at 800-826-0826 or www.uoaa.org.

Possible Challenges

Consider the following challenges that other people have faced:

"I could never learn to change this colostomy pouch."

Learning to deal with a colostomy can be overwhelming. Acknowledge that it seems difficult, but reassure the person that others have learned how and that you will be there to help him or her in any way you can. Nurses and therapists who are specialists in colostomy care can be valuable sources of support and information as the person adjusts to the ostomy.

"My husband won't let me help with his ostomy. He says it is too embarrassing. But he clearly needs help since he is having problems."

Nurses and therapists who specialize in ostomy care are skilled in dealing with feelings of embarrassment. Ask one of them for advice. It may be helpful for him to meet with the specialist who can explain that he does need help.

"My wife won't wear her prosthesis. She says it is uncomfortable, but she doesn't want to bother the doctor or nurse."

Her doctors and nurses want her to have the best care, and this care includes having a prosthesis that is comfortable and practical for her to use. Explain that her health care team would want her to tell them about her problems. If necessary, talk to the nurse yourself, and the nurse can encourage your wife to persist until she has a comfortable prosthesis.

Carrying Out and Adjusting Your Plan

Think of other challenges that could interfere with carrying out your plan. What additional roadblocks could get in the way of following the recommendations in this chapter? Develop plans for getting around challenges by using the COPE ideas discussed in the introduction.

It can take time for the person to accept that an ostomy or prosthesis is a part of life. Being patient and supportive is important. It also takes time to learn how to manage these new body parts. You should keep informed about what needs to be done, and be available whenever the person asks for help. Your goal is to help make the ostomy or prosthesis a normal part of the person's life.

If problems adjusting to the new body part continue and don't seem to be getting better, encourage the person with cancer to talk to the doctor or nurse. Ask for a referral to a professional who specializes in helping people cope with ostomies or prostheses. If the person remains very upset about the changes, suggest talking to a mental health professional. See the chapter on depression for more information on how to recognize severe emotional distress and how to manage this problem.

CHAPTER TWENTY-SIX

Sexual Issues

Sex is a very sensitive subject, and coping with sexual problems requires careful thought and planning on the part of both partners. Since sexual problems are rarely emergencies, there is time to plan and deal with the problems sensitively. The goal is for the person with cancer and his or her sexual partner to work together.

Cancer and cancer treatments can affect a person's sexual desire, behavior, and pleasure, and adjusting to those changes is an important part of coping with the illness. It is important for the person with cancer and his or her partner to understand why sexual changes are happening, to know what to expect, and to know what they can do to deal with or adjust to those changes.

Sexual problems that occur during or after cancer treatment can have physical causes, emotional causes, or both. Physically, most cancer treatments do not injure parts of the body that give orgasms or sexual enjoyment. Exceptions include some treatments that affect the brain or spinal cord, certain surgeries, such as mastectomy (removal of a breast) or orchiectomy (removal of one or both testicles), medicines that change normal hormone balance, and radiation therapy to the lower abdominal or genital areas. Intercourse or sexual intimacy may be affected by these treatments, but people can still have feelings of pleasure. Side effects of treatments, such as pain, nausea, or fatigue, can also affect or reduce sexual pleasure. Finally, changes in the way a man or woman feels about his or her personal attractiveness can have an effect.

Adjusting to Sexual Changes

Talk over feelings or concerns. It is important for the person with cancer to discuss any fears or questions with his or her sexual partner. Talking about sexual matters with a close friend or medical professional can also help.

Plan periods of time for intimacy when you will not be interrupted. Privacy is important for relaxation and sexual pleasure. Planning for uninterrupted time might be difficult, but it will make it easier to give the time and attention to intimacy that is needed.

A great deal of pleasure comes from touching and being held. Sexual intimacy can be achieved without intercourse, without orgasms, and without erections or ejaculation. Being held and touched is an important part of all sexual intimacy and may be even more important when other sexual activities are restricted. Intimacy can be expressed by holding hands, putting an arm around the waist or shoulders, rubbing the back or arms and legs, and any other type of touching. Touch brings comfort and security.

When to Get Professional Help

Talk to the doctor or nurse if any of the following conditions exist:

- *Pain during intercourse.* Any pain with intercourse is a reason to talk to the doctor. Women should report painful intercourse to the gynecologist and ask for advice about trying other positions or continuing intercourse. If a gynecologist has not been involved in the person's care, report the pain to the surgeon or doctor in charge, who can make a referral to a gynecologist. Men should report pain during intercourse and any redness on or unusual discharge from the penis. Radiation therapy to the abdominal or pelvic area can cause pain during intercourse for men and women. If the person has pain after radiation therapy, discuss this issue with the radiation oncologist.

- *Uncertainty about when it is okay to have intercourse.* Sometimes people are reluctant to talk about their sexual activities; however, it is best to be open and to ask the doctor or nurse about when it is okay to resume intercourse. It is also important to ask about symptoms that may be a sign to stop intercourse.

- *Nervousness about sex (for the person or his or her partner).* Sometimes the person's partner may want to resume sexual activity but may be afraid of hurting the person with cancer, spreading the cancer, or even getting cancer themselves. The person who has gone through cancer may be fearful that sex will be painful or unenjoyable. Talking about these concerns with doctors and nurses can be helpful. Cancer is not contagious, and it will not spread through sexual activity.

- *Concern because of lack of interest in sex.* If either of you is concerned about having little interest in sex, discussing the problem with a doctor or nurse can help. Health care professionals can explain the causes and when sexual interest may be expected to return.

- *Inability or unwillingness to talk about changes in sexual activities or feelings, even when asked.* Talking about sexual issues can be difficult, especially if the person with cancer has not talked openly about sex in the past, feels unattractive, or does not want to admit to having sexual problems.

- ***Concerns about pregnancy and reproductive issues.*** Pregnancy usually must be avoided during chemotherapy, so effective birth control is necessary. If the person is concerned about fertility and the possible effects of treatment, speak with the health care team before treatment begins.

Not all professionals will be knowledgeable about these issues; if the first professional you talk to can't help, keep looking. Ask for a referral to a professional counselor who has experience helping people with sexual issues.

What You Can Do

As a partner, you can help deal with sexual issues by following these guidelines:

- **Understand the sexual effects of cancer and cancer treatments and what can be done to deal with those effects.**
- **Help the person with cancer prevent infections from sexual contact.**
- **Be open to changes in sexual routines and behaviors.**

Understand the Sexual Side Effects of Cancer and Cancer Treatment

Sexual side effects will differ for men and women.

Understand sexual side effects for women with cancer.

Treatments and surgery in the pelvic or abdominal areas can change sexual responses or affect a woman's willingness to be touched intimately. Women who have had hysterectomies, urinary surgery, or surgery that increases the likelihood of urine leaking can benefit from these suggestions:

- ***Empty the bladder before intercourse or sexual intimacy.***
  Muscles around the opening to the vagina may have been weakened by surgery. The opening to the tube that carries urine out of the body may also have been weakened. Emptying the bladder before sexual touching or intercourse decreases the chance of urine leaking out. If the woman's urinary system has been injured after surgery or because of cancer, she may need to insert a catheter to remove urine from the bladder. Feelings of fullness in the bladder can interfere with feelings of sexual relaxation and pleasure.
- ***Lubricate the vagina with a water-based gel before sexual activity.***
  Vaginal dryness can be caused by some cancer treatments, such as some chemotherapy regimens, radiation treatment, and surgery. Vaginal dryness can also happen because of

aging or general worry about having sex. Dryness can be treated by lubricating the vagina with a water-based gel before sexual activity. Some brands can be used a few times during the week to help soften and moisturize the vagina and outside skin. These brands do not have to be used every day or every time before intercourse. For best results, avoid petroleum jelly and look in the pharmacy for a gel that does not have an alcohol base. Ask the pharmacist for help.

- ***If the person is taking hormones, learn what changes to expect in sexual feelings and responses and how long these changes will last.***

  Sometimes, anti-estrogens are prescribed to reduce the risk of breast cancer recurrence. These anti-estrogens may have side effects. Find out when side effects may appear and how long they will last. Ask how anti-estrogens may affect vaginal wetness or feelings of desire and excitement. The doctor or nurse can tell you what side effects to expect.

- ***If the person is undergoing chemotherapy or radiation treatment, learn what changes to expect in sexual feelings and responses and how long these changes will last.***

  Some chemotherapy medicines and radiation treatments cause changes in vaginal wetness and in normal sexual responses. Ask the nurse or doctor about changes caused by these types of cancer treatment.

- ***Find out whether the cancer treatment will cause infertility.***

  Some cancer surgeries or treatments can cause female infertility. For example, when the ovaries or uterus are removed, a woman can no longer have a child. High-dose radiation can also result in infertility.

- ***Talk to someone who has had similar experiences.***

  Call your American Cancer Society at **800-227-2345** and ask about Reach to Recovery® if the person has had a mastectomy, lumpectomy, or postmastectomy reconstruction for breast cancer. Reach to Recovery volunteers can answer questions about sexuality, feeling attractive, and sexual activities. A volunteer who has had a similar experience with breast cancer, surgery, and treatment can be assigned to the person. These volunteers often visit the person in the hospital and at home. They can also demonstrate arm exercises to do after surgery; explain what to expect during the healing process; and discuss dressing, bras, and breast prostheses.

➠ Understand sexual side effects for men with cancer.

Encourage men with cancer to do the following:

- ***Ask whether "dry orgasms" will happen.***

  When a man experiences the sensations of orgasm but does not ejaculate, it is called a "dry orgasm." Certain surgeries and treatments cause more sex-related nerve and blood

238

vessel damage than others. Nerve and blood vessel damage near the penis, prostate, or in the pelvic area can change the way men experience desire, erections, and orgasms. Such injuries can also affect whether men continue to ejaculate.

- *If the man might want to father children in the future, find out whether banking sperm is an option before treatment begins.*
  Some cancer surgeries and treatments, such as removal of the testicles or high-dose radiation therapy in the genital area, result in sterility. If either of you are concerned about sterility, ask the doctor about banking sperm, especially if there is even a slight possibility that he may want to become a father. Sperm is collected by the man before the surgery or treatment and frozen (or "banked") for future use. That sperm can later be implanted in a woman through artificial insemination.

- *Find out whether the person will be able to take supplemental hormones if cancer treatment has lowered testosterone levels.*
  The level of testosterone sometimes falls after cancer surgery or treatments. A low testosterone level can cause problems with erections and lower sexual desire. Some men are able to take supplemental testosterone. In the case of prostate cancer, however, supplemental male hormones are not given because they can speed up the growth of the prostate cancer.

- *If the person is taking the synthetic estrogen diethylstilbestrol (DES), ask about any side effects.*
  Be sure to ask about the expected side effects of DES and when they will appear, including how DES may change sexual responses, such as erections or feelings of desire.

- *Ask about penile implants and other options.*
  Erections may be a problem after cancer treatment or surgery. Penile implants or prostheses can be options for men who want more success with erections. Some create a permanent or semirigid erection that can be hidden under clothes. Other implants are inflatable, which gives the man more control over when to have an erection. In this case, a small pump is placed under the skin, and the man pushes the pump several times to cause an erection. Other types of implants and options are also available. Surgeons and urologists can discuss the pros and cons of each option with the person with cancer and his sexual partner.

Help the Person with Cancer Prevent Infection from Sexual Contact

Infections can be caused by sexual contact when the person's immune system is functioning poorly as a result of chemotherapy or radiation treatment. Encourage the person to do the following to prevent infections:

➠ **Wash hands before and after sexual contact and after using the bathroom.**

Thorough hand washing is the most important way to prevent infection caused by touching the genitals.

➠ **Urinate after sex.**

Urinating after sex rinses the genital area of bacteria that may cause infection. After sexual activity, new bacteria are left near the urinary tract. Should the immune system be impaired, these bacteria can lead to infection in the urinary tract or elsewhere. Ask the doctor whether the person is at increased risk for infection caused by sexual contact.

➠ **Avoid sexual contact with people who may have infections or transmissible diseases.**

This includes all infectious diseases, from colds to sexually transmitted diseases, including acquired immunodeficiency syndrome (AIDS). Condoms can help prevent the spread of infectious diseases, but they are not 100 percent effective for all infections. If condoms are used, use a water-based lubricant on the outside of the condom. Do not use oil-based lubricants, such as petroleum jelly, shortening, mineral oil, massage oils, or body lotions, since they can cause the condom to break.

➠ **Clean the rectum thoroughly after bowel movements.**

Infections are easily spread from bacteria around the anus to the opening of the vagina or penis. The best way to prevent infection is to gently wash the anus and surrounding skin with warm water and soap.

Be Open to Changes in Sexual Routines and Behaviors

After cancer treatment, some sexual behaviors may need to be changed or be more gentle. Intimate moments between a couple can be very comforting and reassuring, as well as being pleasurable. Experimentation is key. Try to do what you can to help your partner experience sexual closeness.

➠ **Use a pillow under the hips.**

A pillow can cushion the weight of one person on another and ease any discomfort. It also raises the hips, which can help with penetration.

➠ **Offer gentle masturbation.**

Help the person with cancer experience arousal or orgasm by gently stroking him or her while he or she is lying in a comfortable position.

▸ **Set the mood.**

Recreate a setting from the past in which you were intimate as a couple. Even lying together and holding each other in a quiet setting can bring back feelings of sexual closeness.

Possible Challenges

Here are challenges other people have faced in dealing with sexual problems from cancer:

"Who would think of sex at a time like this?"

Sexual feelings and thoughts can happen anytime, and it is normal to have them. They may be caused by a need to be close and to feel loved, secure, and accepted. Sexual activities may also distract a person from worries.

"He is concerned about sex, but he doesn't want to talk about it."

You can mention to the doctor that he is concerned about sex, and the doctor can raise the issue when talking with him. You can also ask about whether a sex therapist works in your area. Sex therapists are professionals who specialize in helping people learn or relearn how to enjoy sexual contact. Often their fees are covered by insurance if the visits are ordered by a doctor. Often only a few visits are needed to learn about what to do and how to cope with changes in sexual life.

"I am afraid to have intercourse or do anything like we used to do."

It may take time to get comfortable again with touching or having intercourse. Talk with a trusted health care professional. He or she will understand your concerns and help you with ideas on how to give and receive sexual pleasure. No matter how old a person is, being touched and held are important ways to show affection and feel comforted, even if you must postpone or give up intercourse.

Carrying Out and Adjusting Your Plan

Think of other challenges that could interfere with carrying out your plan to deal with sexual issues. What additional roadblocks could get in the way of following the recommendations in this chapter? Will the person with cancer be willing to discuss these issues? How will you explain your needs to counselors or therapists? Develop plans for getting around these challenges by using the COPE ideas discussed in the introduction.

Sex is a sensitive subject for most people. Think carefully about how to discuss the subject with the person with cancer. Be patient and let the person with cancer move at a pace that is comfortable for him or her. Health professionals can be very helpful. They are often skilled in raising and discussing sexual matters; however, not all professionals are skilled or knowledgeable in sexual issues. Therefore, if the first professional you talk with is not helpful, persist until you find a knowledgeable professional who can help with these issues.

For more information about fertility and cancer or other topics related to sexuality and cancer, visit **cancer.org** or call **800-227-2345**.

Part V

Transitioning from Curing to Caring

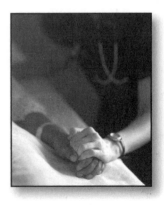

TODAY, MORE PEOPLE THAN EVER BEFORE GO ON TO RECOVER FROM THEIR CANCER. Many people who receive a cancer diagnosis will go on to live long and productive lives. For some people with cancer, however, the focus of care will eventually shift toward making the person comfortable for the time that remains. This can be a time when the person with advanced cancer and his or her caregivers, family, and friends face many new challenges. It is the time when ensuring quality of life—and not length of life—is the primary goal of medical care and treatment and also, ideally, the primary goal of caregivers and family members.

It can be very difficult to talk about illness and dying. It is important, however, for the person with cancer and for you as the caregiver to be able to come to terms with what is happening. The information in these two chapters is written to help the person with cancer, the caregiver, and family and friends cope with the final stages of the person's illness.

For more information about end-of-life care, contact the American Cancer Society at **800-227-2345** or visit the Web site at **cancer.org**.

CHAPTER TWENTY-SEVEN

Palliative Care and the Caregiver

Care that is focused not on curing the disease, but on preventing, reducing, or relieving the symptoms of the disease, is called palliative care. Whereas curative treatment is intended to alter the course of the disease, the goal of palliative care is to achieve the best possible quality of life for the person with cancer. This can mean relieving suffering, controlling pain and symptoms, and enabling the patient to live as normal a life as possible.

Good palliative care is more than just an emphasis on symptom management and quality of life; it is also an attitude toward patient care. Palliative care means treating and caring for the whole person, including the body, mind, and spirit. It means looking at the person with cancer in context—not only as a patient with a disease and symptoms, but as a husband, wife, or partner; father or mother; son or daughter; neighbor; friend; or coworker. Respect for the person's culture, beliefs, and values are essential components. The goal of palliative care is for people to have the best possible quality of life throughout their illness, so that they can enjoy every day to the fullest.

As the disease advances, the number and intensity of symptoms a person with cancer experiences tend to increase. At this stage, the health care team tries to relieve pain and other discomfort and provide care in a way that is consistent with their expressed desires. Palliative care does not hasten or postpone death. Rather, its aim is for people in the end stages of life to have the opportunity to make choices, actively participate in their care, and say and do what matters most to them, even in their final moments.

Hospice Care

Hospice care programs provide supportive care for the patient and the family in the final stages of disease—that is, the last months, weeks, or days of life. Hospice care can be provided in the home, in hospitals that have hospice units, or in free-standing hospice facilities. Hospice care seeks to make the patient as comfortable as possible, relieve symptoms, and help the patient and family have the best possible quality of life. Services are usually covered by insurance and Medicare.

Some people prefer to die at home, while others feel better in a hospital setting. Most often, hospice care takes place in a person's home, and while intermittent nursing care is available, most responsibility still falls to family or other caregivers. In hospice programs, a team of professionals visit the home to help the family keep the person comfortable and to give physical care, such as administering pain medicine, bathing, and helping with toileting. Hospice workers are skilled in controlling pain and in managing symptoms caused by advanced cancer. They can also give emotional and spiritual support to the person with cancer and the family, if wanted. Volunteers may help by coming to the home to give the family a chance to rest.

When making choices about end-of-life care and considering the importance of the person being at home in his or her final days, it is important to recognize the major role that the family or other caregivers will have in caring for the person at home. There are no right or wrong choices, only personal ones that are best for you and your family. Hospice works with the family to provide care, and to meet the physical, functional, emotional, and spiritual needs of the patient. Accepting death is central to the hospice approach, although the focus is on caring for and supporting the patient, helping him or her to live as fully as possible until the end of life.

Physicians may not raise the topic of the transition to palliative care or openly discuss how much time a person has left unless asked directly about the prognosis. Asking specific questions can help, because it encourages openness and may facilitate planning for the remaining time. Doctors are rarely able to pinpoint the amount of time remaining in a person's life. Some people survive longer than predicted, and some die more quickly than expected. Hospice care is designed to care for people with less than six months to live.

To find hospice care in your community, consult qualified health care professionals. Ask a doctor, nurse, or social worker to give you a list of local hospice services. These services may also be listed in the yellow pages of the telephone book. Agencies that will know about hospice care in your community include the Area Office on Aging, the local Visiting Nurse Association, your state's home care association, and the National Hospice and Palliative Care Association. See the resource guide at the end of this book for national contact information. State and local agencies are listed in the white and blue pages of your telephone book. You can also contact your American Cancer Society at **800-227-2345** or visit **cancer.org** to learn about hospice programs near you.

The Role of the Caregiver

It can be difficult to balance the responsibilities of caregiving with the demands and needs of your own life. Research shows that family caregivers are at increased risk for fatigue, physical illness, and emotional distress. Families may bear an additional financial burden when caring for a family member who is ill. Families face intense emotional feelings and potential stressors when confronted with the impending loss of a loved one. Taking care of someone at the end of his or her life will require continuity of care, a good plan, and lots of help. Knowing what to expect in these final months, days, and hours, and knowing what you can do to give the best possible care can help lessen the burden.

Your role as a giver of care, love, and support will be increasingly important during this last phase of his or her illness. As you move through these remaining months, days, and hours, the number of tasks you take on may become greater or the tasks themselves may become more difficult. As you contemplate these challenges, know that there are many things you can do to ensure that you and the person for whom you are caring can make the most of the time that remains. You can improve both the physical comfort and emotional well-being of the person with cancer.

Physical Comfort

Providing physical comfort will mostly mean controlling, managing, or reducing distressing symptoms from treatment, the cancer, or other diseases. Take care of the symptoms that appear. They not only diminish the overall sense of well-being, but they can lead to psychological changes such as depression. Symptom management means reporting changes to the health care team and paying attention to things like pain, fatigue, and loss of appetite. Toward the end of life, people with advancing cancer may become more introspective and sleep with greater frequency or for longer periods. This final period can also be marked by loss of function, acute weight loss, decreased ability to eat and drink, drowsiness, and, in some cases, confusion and delusional behavior. Make sure to discuss what steps you are taking to address these symptoms with the health care professionals to ensure the most appropriate course of treatment.

Emotional Well-being

The declining physical health of the person with cancer may be an opportunity for him or her (and for you) to strengthen emotional bonds. Attending to the emotional needs and psychological well-being of the person with cancer and following your own instincts about the same things are important parts of caring for someone nearing the end of life. Consider how to provide opportunities for self-expression and reminiscing, planning for end of life, confirming social connections, and grieving.

➡ Allow opportunities for self-expression.
Allow yourself and the person with cancer to talk openly about your feelings, and encourage open discussion of topics you need to plan together. It is important for those going through such

a stressful experience to feel free to share whatever feelings and ideas they have, without reproach or guilt. You and the person with cancer will no doubt experience a broad range of emotions. It is healthy to experience laughter and sadness and to reflect on the past and the value of long-term relationships. You may begin to talk about the sense of loss and other feelings that arise as the person nears the end of his or her life. As the caregiver, it is important for you to stay active and verbally engage with other people. Caregivers who isolate themselves physically and emotionally are at greater risk for personal illness and unresolved grief that lasts for long periods.

Use the time you have with the person to think about and reflect on life. You may want to look through old photographs together or look at videos of family gatherings. The person may enjoy looking through old high school or college yearbooks. Reflecting on a life well lived can be an important part of coming to terms with death—for both the caregiver and the person with cancer.

⮞ Confirm social connections.

Maintain as many connections with friends, family, and neighbors as possible during this time. Try to keep people informed about the progression of the person's illness. The network of family and friends can be an invaluable source of support. Social interaction also provides support for you as a caregiver, making it easier for you to carry the weight of your caring tasks. Remember that people will react differently; some will draw closer, whereas others may not be able to visit or interact with you during this period. Some people may pull away because of their own inability to deal with the disease, the situation, or because they do not know exactly what to say or how to help.

⮞ Plan for the end of life.

Encourage the person to think about his or her final days and begin the process of saying goodbye. Some people take advantage of the time they have left to plan and thank friends and family and say goodbye. Talk to the person about how he or she would like to be remembered. There may be things the person would like acknowledged about his or her life in a memorial service or eulogy.

It is important that the person talk with family about his or her preferences in the face of medical emergencies, life-saving interventions, and his or her desire to use resuscitation. These are not easy topics to discuss or broach, but they are essential for any family facing the final months, weeks, or days of life. Encourage the person with advanced cancer to sign a living will or advanced directive. The person should choose one or more people to act as representatives and decision makers in the event that he or she cannot make decisions about medical treatment. Problems can arise if a living will has not been executed and the person becomes unable to make decisions about his or her care.

Another part of planning for end of life can mean reflecting on one's legacy. A legacy is often thought of as "leaving a mark" on the family and the world. A legacy does not have to be financial, although it could be. Some people leave a box of items for young children to open at a later date. Others leave written messages, either in the form of letters to loved ones or notes hidden in strategic locations to be found by a specific person. Notes left in favorite books or hidden within favorite items could be at risk of never being found, so the location should be carefully considered.

A measure of peace and acceptance is required to be able to transcend physical problems and contemplate the legacy of a life. Everyone brings different life experiences, strengths, and capacity for coping with stress to this final stage of life. For some people, the passage through the end of life is rapid, with little time for preparation and reflection. For many people with cancer, there is time to prepare and consider the legacy one wishes to leave behind. Caregivers should do all they can to assist in this process.

⚏➡ Plan funeral and memorial services.

Talk to the person in advance about his or her preferences for what happens after he or she dies. Some people want a simple memorial and are happy to let a loved one or caregiver make plans. Others may want to be more actively involved in planning, whether that means specifying who should read a eulogy or speak, deciding where the memorial will take place, and choosing a time of day for the service. Some people choose the music they would like for the service. Some people use the memorial service as an opportunity to celebrate a life, whereas others use the time to simply share the mourning process.

The caregiver or loved one can play an important role in this planning by encouraging the person with cancer to talk about his or her preferences, recording these wishes, and ensuring they are acted upon after his or her death.

In addition to planning a memorial service, you will need to consider the practical topic of final disposition of bodily remains. If the person's religion mandates certain rituals, they should be respected and followed as meticulously as possible. Make certain that you or someone close to you knows the person's preferences. They can be included as part of a will, though many people simply relate this information verbally. It can be a relief for you to know ahead of time how these details should be handled. It also is a relief to be able to carry out final requests and feel satisfied that you fulfilled the person's wishes.

Grieving

Allow yourself to grieve. Don't feel as though you need to postpone grieving until after the person's death. Grieving now can help you acknowledge the reality of the situation and can provide a healthy outlet for the many complex emotions you and the person you care about are likely experiencing.

The process of grieving may have started when cancer was first diagnosed. As the person's death approaches, you are likely to experience something called anticipatory grief. During this process, which precedes the person's actual death, you begin to realize the inevitability of this loss and you begin to think about how life will change after his or her passing. You should not be surprised by this response; these feelings are natural and acceptable. In fact, you can learn a great deal about grief during this time. The behaviors you demonstrate during anticipatory grief may be good predictors of how you will respond after the person's death.

The end of life represents significant loss—loss of life, loss of important relationships, and loss of opportunity. These losses can generate strong emotions, including grief, anger, and frustration, and it is important that you each feel able to express those emotions. Some people may try to repress their feelings or shield the person with cancer from them. In the long run, however, openness often accomplishes more than denial. Avoiding the topic of impending death can be isolating.

Denial and disbelief may be common emotions for both people with advanced cancer and their families, but lasting denial diminishes the capacity to deal with treatment, financial and legal plans, and even discussion of preferences for funeral arrangements. Not surprisingly, as many as one in four people with advanced cancer demonstrate moderate to severe denial. Grief and other emotions are a natural part of the process of coming to terms with impending death. Denial may delay coming to terms with the death.

On the other hand, denial can be a protective coping mechanism and, in that regard, it can be helpful *to an extent*. Also, just because a person who is seriously ill does not want to dwell upon or talk about his or her impending death does not mean the person is in denial. Accepting death can bring peace and comfort. Sometimes it is a relief to know that the person with cancer will be released from further discomfort or pain.

CHAPTER TWENTY-EIGHT

Patient Symptoms and How to Help

When caring for a loved one who has advanced cancer, you may be with him or her at the time of death. The following is intended to help with some of the anxiety that surrounds the end of life by looking at the process of dying.

This section describes some signs that death may be close. Not all of the following symptoms will happen, but it may be comforting to know about them. People often use this time to gather the family to say goodbye. They may take turns with the person, holding hands, talking, or just sitting quietly. It can also be a time to perform any religious rituals or other activities the person wants before death. It is a chance for family and friends to express their love and appreciation for the person and for each other.

It is important to have a plan for what to do after death, so that the family knows what to do during this very emotional time. If the person is in hospice, the hospice nurse and social worker will help you. If the person is not in hospice, talk with your doctor about it so that you will know what to do at the time of death.

In addition to the following descriptions, see also figure 28.1 for a list of possible changes in body function and what you can do about them.

These are some of the signs the person is nearing death:
- Profound weakness—usually the person cannot get out of bed and has trouble moving around in bed.
- The person needs help with nearly everything he or she does.
- There is less and less interest in food, often with very little food and fluid intake for days.
- Drowsiness will increase—the person may doze or sleep much of the time if pain is relieved. He or she may be hard to rouse or wake.

- The person may be restless and pick or pull at bed linens. Anxiety, fear, restlessness, and loneliness may worsen at night.
- The person cannot concentrate or has a short attention span. He or she is confused about time, place, or people.
- Swallowing pills and medicines is difficult.
- He or she has a limited ability to cooperate with caregivers.

Possible Changes in Body Function

- The person will be weak.
- He or she has trouble moving around in bed and may not be able to get out of bed.
- The person cannot change positions without help.
- Swallowing food, medicines, or even liquids will be difficult.
- There may be sudden involuntary movement of muscles, jerking of hands, arms, legs, or face.

⫸ What caregivers can do

As the caregiver, there are several things you can do to increase the person's comfort. Help him or her turn and change positions every hour or two. Try to speak in a calm, quiet voice and avoid sudden noises or movements so that you don't startle the person. If the person is having trouble swallowing pain medicines, ask the doctor or hospice nurse about liquid pain medicines or the pain patch. If the person is having trouble swallowing, avoid giving him or her solid foods. Give ice chips or sips of liquid through a straw. Do not push fluids, however. Near the end of life, some dehydration is normal and is more comfortable for the patient. It may also make the person more comfortable for you to apply cool, moist washcloths to the person's head, face, and body.

Possible Changes in Consciousness

- The person sleeps more during the day and is hard to wake or rouse from sleep.
- The person is confused about time, place, or people. He or she may talk about things unrelated to the events or people present.
- He or she is restless and may pick or pull at bed linens. Restlessness, anxiety, fear, and loneliness may be worse at night.
- After a period of sleepiness and confusion, the person may have a short time when he or she is mentally clear before going back into a semiconscious state.

⫸ What caregivers can do

Plan your time with the person for when he or she is most alert or during the night when your presence may be comforting. When talking with the person, remind him or her who you are and what day and time it is. Use calm, confident, gentle tones to reduce the chances of startling or frightening the person. Touching, caressing, holding, and rocking the person are usually helpful and comforting.

Continue the person's pain medicines up to the end of life. If the person is very restless, try to find out whether he or she is having pain. If it appears so, give "breakthrough" pain medicines as prescribed, or check with the doctor or hospice nurse, if needed.

Even if the person is semiconscious, he or she can often still hear, even though he or she is unable to respond. Words of love and support may still be understood and appreciated. Some people are unconscious for hours or even days before death, whereas others remain clear and alert up to the last few moments.

Possible Changes in Metabolism

- The person has less interest in and need for food and drink.
- His or her mouth may dry out. (See the section on possible changes in secretions below.)
- The person may no longer need some of his or her medicines, such as vitamins, chemotherapy, replacement hormones, blood pressure medicines, and diuretics, unless they help make the person more comfortable.

⓲➤ What caregivers can do

Ice chips, water, or juice can be given as requested but should be stopped if the person has difficulty swallowing. Because the person no longer needs nourishment, solid food should not be given unless the person requests it.

Check with the doctor to see which medicines can be stopped. Medicines for pain, nausea, fever, seizures, or anxiety should be continued to keep the person comfortable.

Care of the person's mouth is important. Apply lubricant or petroleum jelly (Vaseline) to the person's lips to prevent drying. Ice chips from a spoon or sips of water or juice from a straw may be enough for the person.

Possible Changes in Secretions

- Mucus in the mouth may collect in the back of the throat. This can be a very distressing sound to hear but doesn't usually cause discomfort to the person.
- Secretions may thicken because of lower fluid intake and build up because the person cannot cough.

⓲➤ What caregivers can do

If mouth secretions increase, keep them loose by adding humidity to the room with a cool mist humidifier. If the person can swallow, ice chips or sips of liquid through a straw may thin the secretions. Change the person's position—turning him or her to the side may help secretions drain from the mouth. Continue to clean the person's teeth with a soft toothbrush or soft foam mouth swabs. Certain medicines may help the person—ask your hospice or home care nurse.

Possible Changes in Circulation and Temperature

- The person's arms and legs may feel cool to the touch as circulation slows down.
- The skin of the person's arms, legs, hands, and feet may darken in color and appear mottled.
- Other areas of the body may become either darker or more pale.
- His or her skin may feel cold and either dry or damp.
- The person's heart rate may become fast, faint, or irregular.
- The person's blood pressure may get lower and become hard to hear.

➡ **What caregivers can do**

Keep the person warm with blankets or light bed coverings. Avoid using electric blankets or heating pads.

Possible Changes in Senses and Perception

- The person's vision may become blurry or dim.
- His or her hearing may decrease, but most people are able to hear you even after they can no longer speak.

➡ **What caregivers can do**

- Leave indirect lights on as vision decreases. Never assume the person cannot hear you.
- Continue to speak with and touch the person to reassure him or her of your presence. Your words of affection and support are likely to be understood and appreciated.

Possible Changes in Breathing

- Breathing may speed up and slow down because of lower blood circulation and buildup of waste products in the body.
- Mucus in the back of the person's throat may cause rattling or gurgling with each breath.
- The person may not breathe for periods of ten to thirty seconds.

IIII➡ **What caregivers can do**

Put the person on his or her back or slightly to one side. Raising the person's head may give him or her some relief. You can try using pillows to prop the person's head and chest at an angle or raising the head of the hospital bed. Any position that seems to make breathing easier is okay, including sitting up with good support. A small person may be more comfortable in your arms.

Oxygen may help some people, but not all. Medications can be given if breathing becomes uncomfortable for the person with cancer.

Although rattling and gurgling sounds may be distressing to hear, they do not usually indicate any discomfort for the person with cancer. Medications can be given to dry up excessive secretions if this becomes a problem.

Possible Changes in Elimination

- Amounts of urine may decrease and may be darker in color.
- When death is near, the person may lose control of urine and stool.

IIII➡ **What caregivers can do**

- Pad the bed beneath the person with layers of disposable waterproof pads.
- If the person has a catheter, the home health care nurse will teach you to take care of it.

When death does occur, breathing stops and the person's blood pressure cannot be heard. The pulse will stop, and the eyes will stop moving and may stay open. The pupils of the eyes will stay large, even in bright light. Control of the bowels and bladder is lost as the muscles relax.

After death, it is okay to sit with the person for a while. There is no rush to get anything done right away. Many families find this is an important time to talk or pray together and reconfirm their love for each other and for the person who has passed away.

If the person dies in the home, caregivers are responsible for calling the proper people. Regulations or laws about who must be notified and how the body should be removed differ from one community to another. Your doctor or nurse can get this information for you. If you have a hospice or home care agency involved, call them. If you have completed funeral arrangements, calling the funeral director and doctor is usually all you have to do.

Figure 28.1. Signs and Symptoms of Approaching Death

	POSSIBLE CHANGES
BODY FUNCTION	• Increased periods of sleep during the day • Difficulty waking from sleep • Confusion about time, place, or people • Restlessness or picking or pulling at bed linen • Increased anxiety, restlessness, fear, and loneliness at night • Less desire for food and drink
SECRETIONS	• More mucus in the mouth that collects in the back of the throat, causing a distressing sound sometimes called a "death rattle" • More thick secretions due to less fluid intake and the inability to cough
CIRCULATION	• Cooling of arms and legs • Deepening of color and mottling of skin of arms, legs, hands, and feet • Dusky, pale skin in other areas of the body
SENSORY PERCEPTION	• Blurred or dimmed vision • Decreased hearing, though most people are able to hear you even after they can no longer speak
BREATHING	• Irregular breathing caused by poor blood circulation and the buildup of waste products in the body • Periods of no breathing of up to ten to thirty seconds
ELIMINATION	• Decreased urine output • Darkened urine • Loss of bladder and bowel control
DEATH	• Breathing stops • Pulse stops

Source: Advanced Cancer and Palliative Care Treatment Guidelines for Patients, Version I/December 2003. ACS/NCCN. pp. 18–19.

WHAT THE CAREGIVER CAN DO

- Plan to spend time with your loved one when he or she is most alert or during the night, when your presence may be comforting
- Remind your loved one who you are and what day and time it is
- Use a calm, confident voice to reduce chances of startling or frightening the person
- Apply cool, moist washcloths to the person's head, face, and body for comfort

- Keep oral secretions loose by adding humidity to the room with a cool mist humidifier
- Provide ice chips or sips of liquid through a straw if the person is able to swallow; this will thin secretions and relieve thirst and dry mouth
- Change the person's position—turning the person to his or her side may help drain mouth secretions

- Provide blankets if needed or requested
- Avoid use of electric blankets and heating pads

- Leave indirect lights on as vision decreases
- Never assume your loved one cannot hear you
- Continue to speak with and touch your loved one to reassure him or her of your presence

- Raise the person's head and chest with pillows or by raising the hospital bed

- Pad bedding with layers of disposable pads
- Learn how to care for the person's catheter, if necessary

- Call appropriate authorities in accordance with local regulations

APPENDIX A

Cancer Treatments and Clinical Trials

Appendix A gives an overview of different cancer treatments, why they are used, and what to expect before, during, and after, as well as a brief section on clinical trials. This information will help you understand what will be happening to the person for whom you are caring so that you can help him or her get through these experiences.

Use this section as needed. You may not need to read the entire section, only those parts that apply specifically to the person for whom you are caring. For instance, he or she may have surgery followed by chemotherapy, so you may want to read only those parts. Read what feels relevant to your situation. This appendix explores the following types of treatment, as well as clinical trials:

- surgery
- radiation therapy
- chemotherapy
- bone marrow and peripheral blood stem cell transplants
- biotherapy
- targeted therapy
- hormonal therapy

Understanding Informed Consent Before Treatment

Before starting treatment, the person with cancer should feel comfortable that he or she understands what has been explained about the treatment and that all questions have been answered. Before treatment begins, the person will be asked to sign a form giving written permission for the hospital to administer the treatment. This process of receiving and understanding the information and giving permission for treatment to begin is called informed consent. The person's signature acknowledges receipt of this information and a willingness to undergo treatment. This permission should be based on the person's understanding of the following information:

- the treatment recommended by the doctor or oncologist
- the goal of the treatment
- how it will be performed and how long it will take
- the potential risks and benefits of the treatment
- the potential side effects and how they would be treated
- the other options available to the person with cancer

A Second Opinion

When a person receives a cancer diagnosis, getting opinions from at least two doctors can be very helpful in deciding between treatment options. In fact, some insurance companies require that you get a second opinion. You can ask your oncologist or your family doctor for recommendations. Doctors are used to these requests and will respect your right to seek a second opinion. You may also be able to ask your insurance company whether there are other doctors that are covered by your plan.

For more information on any of the treatments discussed in this section, contact the American Cancer Society at **800-227-2345** or visit the Web site, **cancer.org**.

I. Surgery

Surgery is the treatment of disease, injury, or disfigurement by means of an operation. It is the oldest form of treatment for cancer and offers the greatest chance for cure for many cancers. Most people with cancer will have some type of surgery. Surgery may be done for a number of reasons (not all of which involve actual treatment). There are seven different categories of surgery, each with a distinctive goal:

1. **Diagnostic surgery** is used to obtain a tissue sample to confirm whether cancer is present or to identify the specific type of cancer.
2. **Preventive (or prophylactic) surgery** is done to remove an area that is at high risk of becoming cancerous if left untreated.
3. **Staging surgery** is done to determine the extent of the cancer.
4. **Curative surgery** is used to try to remove a tumor when it appears to be localized and there is hope of removing all of the cancer.
5. **Palliative surgery** is done to treat complications of advanced cancer and is not intended as a cure. It can be done to correct a condition that is causing pain or disability, such as clearing a blocked intestine.
6. **Supportive surgery** is used to help with other types of treatment, such as the placement of a catheter under the skin to give chemotherapy treatments at a later time.

7. **Restorative (or reconstructive) surgery** is used to restore a person's appearance or restore the function of an organ or body part. Breast reconstruction after mastectomy is an example of restorative surgery.

Biopsy: Diagnosing Cancer

A *biopsy* is a type of diagnostic surgery—a procedure to remove part or all of a tumor to determine whether it is cancerous. In most cases, some type of biopsy is needed to confirm a diagnosis of cancer.

Some types of biopsies do not require the doctor to make a surgical incision. Small tumor samples can be removed through a hollow needle inserted into the skin or through an endoscope (a flexible lighted tube inserted through a body opening, such as the mouth). Some biopsies can be done in a doctor's office and require only local anesthesia.

Other biopsies require surgical incisions. Minor biopsies of this type, such as those used to remove a suspicious area of skin for testing, can sometimes be done in a doctor's office. More involved biopsies usually need to be done in an operating room. These biopsies typically involve larger surgical incisions or several incisions and may require general anesthesia.

Treating Cancer with Surgery

The type and extent of surgery used to treat cancer varies a great deal, depending on the type of cancer, where it is located, and how advanced it is. Removing some tumors may require only small incisions, whereas the treatment of more advanced tumors may require larger incisions and removal of more body tissue. To reach tumors in the abdomen, surgeons often perform a laparotomy, a long incision through the abdominal wall. Tumors in the chest are often reached with a thoracotomy, an incision through the chest wall.

Recent advances have allowed surgeons to do some operations in the chest or abdomen with much smaller incisions than were used in the past. In *laparoscopic surgery*, the surgeon makes several small cuts in the abdomen and inserts long, thin instruments through them. One of these instruments has a small video camera on the end, which allows the surgeon to see what he or she is doing. A similar operation in the chest is *thoracoscopic surgery*. An even newer approach is *robotic-assisted laparoscopic surgery*. Here, the surgeon sits at a special control panel to precisely move surgical instruments, instead of holding the instruments directly.

These new approaches hold promise in treating cancer while reducing the person's pain and recovery time. But for the most part they are not yet as well proven as standard surgery approaches. These new approaches are also hard to learn and require that surgeons have special training. If you are considering this type of surgery, it is important to find a surgeon with experience performing this type of procedure.

The Surgery Experience

Some parts of the surgery experience are common to most operations. They include preoperative testing and preparation, the surgery itself, and a recovery period.

⫸ Preoperative testing and other preparations

Tests are usually needed in the days or weeks before surgery, especially for major operations. These tests are done to make sure your body can handle surgery and anesthesia. Tests may also be done to better understand your condition and help plan the surgery. You may not need all of these tests (especially if you are having a minor procedure in a doctor's office).

These are the most commonly used preoperative tests:
- *Blood and urine tests* to measure blood counts, the risk of bleeding or infection, and function of the liver and kidneys. The person's blood type may also be determined if there might be a need for blood transfusions during the operation.
- *Chest x-ray* and *electrocardiogram (EKG)* to check lung and heart function
- Other tests as needed, such as a *computed tomography (CT) scan* or *magnetic resonance imaging (MRI)*, to study the size and location of tumors and whether they are involved with nearby structures in the body.

The surgeon will want to know whether there is a history of high blood pressure, heart disease, diabetes, allergies, or other conditions that could affect the surgery. Other specialists may be consulted or other tests may be done if the person has any other conditions that could affect the surgery. The surgeon may also ask the person to stop taking certain medicines, stop smoking or drinking alcohol, improve his or her diet, or actively exercise before surgery.

⫸ Preparing for surgery

Depending on the type of operation, some things may need to be done to prepare for surgery. For example, emptying the digestive tract is important if surgery involves general anesthesia. Preparation may involve not eating or drinking anything, starting the night before the surgery. A laxative or an enema may also be required to make sure the intestines are empty. The health care team will discuss these preparations with the person before surgery.

⫸ Anesthesia during surgery

Anesthesia is the use of drugs to make the body unable to feel pain for a period of time. In some cases, there may be a choice as to which type of anesthesia is used. There are three types of anesthesia:
- *Local anesthesia* is often used for minor surgery, such as a biopsy near the skin's sur-

face. Medicine is injected to numb the local area, but the person stays awake.

- **Regional anesthesia** *(a nerve block)* numbs a larger area of the body. It usually involves injecting medicine into an area around the spinal cord or around nerves in the arms or legs. The person is still awake, though another drug may be given to promote relaxation.

- **General anesthesia** puts the person into a deep sleep for the surgery. Once asleep, an endotracheal (ET) tube is placed in the throat to make it easier for the person to breathe. Vital signs (heart rate, breathing rate, and blood pressure) are closely watched during the surgery. The ET tube is removed once the operation is over.

⮕ Recovery after surgery

With local anesthesia, most people are allowed to go home shortly after the surgery. People who get regional or general anesthesia are taken to a recovery room to be monitored while the effects of the anesthesia wear off. Recovery may take several hours. People waking up from general anesthesia often feel "out of it" for some time.

After surgery, a person may have a catheter in place to drain urine from the bladder into a bag. There may also be a tube or tubes (called drains) coming out of any incision site. Drains allow excess fluid that collects at the surgery site to leave the body. The doctor will likely remove the drains once they stop collecting fluid, usually a few days after the operation.

Eating and drinking are important parts of the recovery process. The stomach and intestines are some of the last parts of the body to recover from the effects of anesthesia. Most people start out with ice chips or water. Signs of stomach and bowel activity need to be present before a person will be allowed to eat.

Once a person is able to eat and get around, plans may be made for going home. Of course, this decision depends upon other factors as well, such as the results of the surgery and tests done afterward. The doctor will want to make sure the person is well enough to be home. Before leaving, the staff will want to be sure the person understands the following information:

- how to care for the wound
- physical signs that might require attention right away
- any physical limitations or other restrictions
- what medicines should be taken and how often
- who to call with questions or problems
- whether anything should be done in terms of rehabilitation
- the date of the next doctor's visit

People often need help at home for a while after surgery. If necessary, a nurse or nurse's aide may be able to visit the person at home for a short while.

Other aspects of recovery may be longer-term in nature. Wounds heal at different rates in different people. Some operations, such as a mastectomy, limb amputation, or ostomy, affect how the body looks and functions and may require learning new ways of doing everyday tasks. Understanding the consequences of the operation beforehand is an important part of helping a person adjust to the changes that surgery will make to the body.

The Risks of Surgery

Medical advances have made modern surgery safer and less invasive than ever before. But there is always a degree of risk involved, no matter how minor the surgery. Before any surgery is done, it is important to understand the risks. Generally, the more complex the surgery, the greater the risk.

ⅢⅢ➤ Possible problems during surgery

Complications during major surgeries are not common, but can include the following:

- bleeding during surgery that may require blood transfusions
- damage to internal organs and blood vessels
- reactions to anesthesia or other medicines
- problems with other organs, such as the lungs, heart, or kidneys. These types of problems are very rare but can happen and can be life-threatening.

ⅢⅢ➤ Possible problems after surgery

There are some fairly common (but not usually life-threatening) problems that occur after surgery:

- *Pain* is probably the most common side effect. Almost everyone has some level of pain after surgery. There are many ways of dealing with surgical pain.
- *Infection* at the site of the wound is another possible problem. Antibiotics are able to prevent or treat most infections.

Other problems are rare but may be more serious:

- *Pneumonia* or other infections
- *Bleeding,* either internally or externally
- *Blood clots* in the deep veins of the legs
- *Slow recovery of other body functions*, such as bowel function if the surgery was near the bowel or abdomen

Long-term side effects depend on the type of procedure and should be discussed with the doctor before surgery.

ⅢⅢ➤ Surgery and metastasis

Does surgery cause cancer to metastasize? In nearly all situations, surgery does not cause cancer to spread, but there are some important exceptions. Doctors who are experienced in taking biopsies of cancers and using surgery as a treatment for cancer are very careful to avoid these situations.

The chances of a needle biopsy causing a cancer to metastasize are extremely low. In the past, larger needles were used for biopsies, and the chance of spread was higher. Most types of cancers can be safely sampled by surgery, but there are a few exceptions, such as certain tumors in the eyes or in the testicles. For these types of cancer, doctors may treat without a biopsy or may recommend removing the entire tumor if it is likely to be cancerous. However, biopsy is the best way to determine whether cancer is present.

One common myth about cancer is that it will spread if it is exposed to air during surgery. Some people may believe this myth because they often feel worse after the operation than they did before. It is normal to feel this way right after surgery. Cancer does not spread because it has been exposed to air.

If you have any concerns about surgery and cancer metastasis, discuss this issue with the people who know your situation best—your surgeon and other members of your health care team.

II. Radiation Therapy

Radiation therapy is the treatment of cancer and other diseases with high-energy particles or waves, such as x-rays, gamma rays, electrons, and protons, that destroy or damage cancer cells. Also known as radiotherapy, x-ray therapy, and irradiation, radiation therapy is one of the most common treatments for cancer and is used in more than half of all cancer cases. It may be given alone, but more often it is combined with other forms of cancer treatment.

Like surgery, radiation therapy is usually a form of localized treatment. It is intended to treat only a specifically targeted part of the body. Radiation therapy is different from forms of systemic treatment, such as chemotherapy, hormonal therapy, or biotherapy, which reach all parts of the body.

Radiation works by damaging the genetic material—the DNA—inside a cell. This damage causes the cell to die when it tries to divide into two new cells. Because cancer cells divide much more frequently than normal cells, they are more likely to be affected by radiation. Although normal cells in the field of treatment are affected by radiation, most recover fully from the effects of treatment.

Radiation therapy can be used in several ways:

- ***To cure or shrink early-stage cancer.*** Some cancers are very sensitive to radiation. Radiation may be used by itself in these cases to make the cancer shrink or go away completely. For other cancers, it may be used before surgery (*neoadjuvant therapy*) to shrink the tumor, after surgery (*adjuvant therapy*) to prevent the cancer from coming back, or during surgery *(intraoperative therapy)* to improve surgical results. It may also be used along with chemotherapy in some situations.

- **To stop cancer from recurring in another area.** If a type of cancer is known to commonly spread to a particular area, the area may be treated, even though no tumors can be seen. For example, some people with lung cancer may receive prophylactic (preventive) radiation to the head because lung cancer often spreads to the brain.
- **To treat symptoms of advanced cancer.** Some cancers may spread too far to be considered curable. But radiation may help to relieve symptoms such as pain, trouble swallowing or breathing, or bowel problems that can be caused by advanced cancer. This use of radiation therapy is often referred to as palliative radiation therapy.

External Radiation Therapy

External radiation (or external-beam radiation) uses a machine that directs radiation at the cancer and some normal surrounding tissue from outside the body. Most people receive external radiation therapy during outpatient visits to a hospital or treatment center.

⯈ Pretreatment and planning

The process of planning external-beam radiation therapy is complex and may take several days to complete. It is one of the most important parts of radiation treatment. The doctor will design a treatment that delivers the strongest possible dose of radiation to the cancer while sparing as much normal tissue as possible, thereby reducing the side effects of treatment.

The first part of treatment planning is called simulation, sometimes referred to as a marking session. The person is asked to lie still on a table while the health care team works out the best treatment position. The team will then mark the radiation field, or treatment port, which is the exact place on the body where the beam of radiation will be aimed. The doctor may use imaging tests such as a CT scan to check the size of the tumor, identify where it is most likely to spread, outline normal tissues in the treatment area, take measurements, and develop the treatment plan.

In a complex procedure called dosimetry, the dosimetrist calculates the radiation dose and the amount of radiation that the surrounding normal tissues would be exposed to in order to deliver the prescribed dose to the cancer. The doctor and dosimetrist work together to determine the amount of radiation to use and the best way to aim it at the cancer. They base this decision on the size of the tumor, how sensitive the tumor is to radiation, and the ability of the normal tissue in the area to withstand the radiation.

⯈ Length of treatment plans

External radiation therapy usually is given five days a week for up to eight weeks. When radiation is used for palliative care, the course of treatment typically lasts for two to three weeks, with radiation given five days a week. These shorter types of schedules are less damaging to normal tissues in the treatment area. Weekend rest breaks allow normal cells to recover. The total dose of radiation and the number of treatments received will depend on the type, size, and location of the person's cancer, his or her general health, and any other treatments being provided.

⫸ Receiving external radiation therapy

External radiation treatments are painless. The experience is like getting a regular x-ray. The actual treatment takes only a few minutes; however, each session can last fifteen to thirty minutes because of the time required to set up the equipment and correctly position the person getting treatment.

Depending on the treatment area, the person may need to get undressed and wear a hospital gown. In the treatment room, the radiation therapist will use the marks on the skin to locate the treatment area. Then the person will sit in a special chair or lie down on a treatment table under the radiation machine.

The radiation therapist may put special shields (or blocks) between the machine and certain parts of the person's body to help protect normal tissues and organs. There might also be plastic or plaster forms to help the person stay in exactly the right place. The person will need to remain very still during the treatment to ensure that the radiation reaches only the area where it is intended and that the same area is treated each time.

Once the person is positioned correctly, the radiation therapist will leave the treatment room before the machine is turned on. The person getting treatment will be watched on a television screen or through a window in a nearby control room but can communicate with the therapist at any time.

The machines used for radiation treatments are very large, and they make noises as they move around to target the treatment area from different angles. Their size and motion may be frightening at first. Remember that the radiation therapist controls the movements of the machines, and they are checked frequently to be sure they are working correctly.

The radiation cannot be seen or heard. If the person feels ill or very uncomfortable during the treatment, he or she should tell the therapist and the machine can be stopped at any time.

There have been some recent advances in radiation therapy that can make it even more effective. Intensity-modulated radiation therapy and three-dimensional conformal radiation therapy make it possible to tailor the radiation therapy to the shape of the tumor and to better spare normal tissues. Proton therapy, a treatment that uses particle beams, is also known for its ability to spare normal tissues, but few centers offer it so far.

Internal Radiation Therapy

Internal radiation therapy, also called brachytherapy or implant therapy, places the source of the radiation as close as possible to the cancer cells. The advantage of brachytherapy is its ability to deliver a high dose of radiation to a small area. It is useful in situations that require a high dose of radiation or a dose that would exceed what normal tissues could tolerate if it was given externally. It is sometimes used for cancers of the head and neck, breast, uterus, thyroid, cervix, and prostate.

Instead of using a large radiation machine, the radioactive material is placed directly into (or as close as possible to) the affected area. The material may be in the form of small pellets, wire, tubes, containers, or even radioactive solutions. These materials may be placed directly into tissues (interstitial therapy), as when treating prostate cancer; placed into nearby body cavities (intracavitary therapy), as when treating cervical cancer; or injected into the bloodstream through an intravenous (IV) line, as when treating thyroid cancer.

⮕ Receiving internal radiation therapy

When internal radiation is given, the placement of these materials can be permanent or temporary:

- *Permanent brachytherapy* involves using small containers, called pellets or seeds, which are about the size of a grain of rice. They are placed directly into tumors using thin, hollow needles. Once in place, the pellets give off low-dose radiation for several weeks or months. Because they are so small and cause little discomfort, they are simply left in place after all of the radioactive material is used.
- *Temporary brachytherapy* involves temporarily placing hollow needles, tubes, or fluid-filled balloons into the area to be treated. Radioactive material can then be inserted for a short period of time and then removed. This process may be repeated over the course of a few days or weeks. Depending on how long the radioactive material is left in place, it may be necessary to stay in a hospital bed and lie fairly still to keep the implant from shifting.

Severe pain or illness is not likely to occur during internal radiation therapy. A person may feel drowsy, weak, or nauseated for a short time because of the anesthesia used while the implant is being placed. Anesthesia is usually not needed to take out the implant. Most implants can be taken out right in the hospital room. If you had to stay in bed during internal radiation therapy, you might have to remain in the hospital an extra day or so after the implant is removed.

Whereas the radiation from brachytherapy generally travels only a short distance, to be safe, doctors often advise taking precautions to make sure others are not exposed to radiation. During temporary brachytherapy, the hospital may require the person to stay in a private room.

Although nurses and other caregivers may not be able to spend a long time in the person's room, they will provide all necessary care.

There may also be limits on visitors while the implant is in place. Most hospitals do not let children or pregnant women visit people who have an implant. Visitors should ask the nurse for specific instructions before entering the hospital room.

The amount of time that an implant is left in place depends on the dose of radioactivity with which the person is treated. The implant may have a low dose rate and be left in place for several days or may have a high dose rate and be removed after a few minutes. Generally, low dose rate implants are left in place between one and seven days.

Once the implant is removed, there is no radioactivity in the body. The doctor will tell the person if physical activity should be limited for a time. Most people are encouraged to resume normal activities, as they feel able. Some people need extra sleep or rest breaks during their first days at home. The area that has been treated may be sore or sensitive for some time after therapy.

If the implant is permanent, the person with cancer may be able to go home that day or may need to stay in a hospital room for a day or two. The implant will lose radioactivity each day.

Follow-up Care

After radiation therapy is finished, it is important to have regular exams to monitor the results of treatment. The radiation oncologist will want to see the person being treated at least once after treatment ends. The doctor who referred the person for radiation therapy will schedule follow-up visits as needed. Follow-up care, in addition to checking the results of treatment, might also include more cancer treatment, rehabilitation, and counseling.

Most people with cancer return to the radiation oncologist for regular follow-up visits. Others are referred back to their original doctor, to a surgeon, or to a medical oncologist. Just as every person with cancer is different, follow-up care varies. The person may find he or she needs extra rest while healthy tissues are rebuilding. The person may need some time to test his or her strength, little by little, and a full schedule may not be advised right away.

III. Chemotherapy

Chemotherapy is one of several treatments that may be used to help people with cancer. Depending on the type and extent (stage) of the cancer, chemotherapy can be used to achieve the following goals:

- to try to cure the cancer
- to help prevent the cancer from coming back after other treatments (such as surgery)
- to shrink tumors so that local treatments, such as surgery, might be more effective

- to help keep advanced cancer from growing or spreading further
- to relieve symptoms caused by the cancer

It is important to know the goal of chemotherapy before starting treatment. If the goal is unclear, ask the doctor. Many different chemotherapy drugs are available, though only certain ones may be useful against specific types of cancer. A single chemotherapy drug can be used to treat cancer, but generally these drugs are more effective when they are combined. Combination chemotherapy uses drugs with different actions to kill more cancer cells and reduces the chance that a person will develop a resistance to one particular drug.

Sometimes, as with some advanced cancers, chemotherapy may be the only treatment a person receives. More often, chemotherapy is used along with other treatments such as surgery or radiation therapy.

Drug Delivery Methods

Chemotherapy can be given in a number of different ways, depending on the type of cancer and the drug or drugs given:

- *By mouth in pill, capsule, or liquid form.* If the person is taking chemotherapy drugs orally at home, it is important to make sure he or she takes the exact dosage that has been prescribed.
- *By injection.* Health professionals can inject chemotherapy agents into a muscle, into a tumor under the skin, or into the skin itself.
- *By intravenous (IV) line or catheter into a vein.* Intravenous administration is the most common way to get chemotherapy. The drug is infused through an IV line, usually on the hand or forearm, but sometimes into a central venous catheter, which is implanted into the chest. The drug may be given either over a few minutes (an "IV push"), as an infusion that lasts up to a few hours, or as a continuous infusion that lasts up to several days. For continuous infusions, the amount of drug given over time is controlled by a small pump, which can be inside or outside the body. This pump allows a person to move around while it is in use.
- *By injection or IV access into other areas.* Chemotherapy drugs can be administered into the spinal fluid (intrathecal), a body cavity like the abdomen (intracavitary), or a large artery (intra-arterial).

Needles can scar or weaken veins after several IV chemotherapy sessions. An alternative to the use of IV lines is to have a catheter put in place. A central venous catheter (CVC) is surgically implanted in the chest, with the end of the catheter either outside the body or just under the skin. It can remain in place for several months to provide access to a large vein. Another option is a long-term catheter placed in the arm, which does not require surgery. Chemotherapy drugs can be injected into these catheters, and blood samples can be drawn from the catheter for tests. There are many different kinds of catheters. Many people discuss this option with their doctors even before starting treatment. Some find out during treatment that they need a catheter because their hand and arm veins are too damaged to complete the planned chemotherapy. If a catheter is placed, it is important to know how to care for it to reduce the risk of infection. Another option is a port, a small, round disc that is placed just under the skin in the area just below the collarbone.

Treatment Schedules

Chemotherapy schedules vary for different people. It may be given once a day, once a week, or even once a month depending on the individual, the type of cancer, and the drugs being used. It is usually given in on-and-off cycles, in which a period of treatment is followed by a rest period. Rest periods allow the body a chance to build healthy new cells and regain strength. Whatever schedule the doctor prescribes, encourage the person to stick with it. Otherwise, the drugs might not have the desired effect. If a treatment session or a dose of medicine is missed, contact the doctor to find out what to do.

The doctor may sometimes delay a treatment if the results of blood tests show the person's body needs more time to recover. The doctor will let the person know what to do during this time and when it is okay to start treatment again.

The length of time chemotherapy is given can also vary. This schedule can depend on the type of cancer, how it responds to treatment, and how well the person is tolerating treatment.

Chemotherapy and Other Medicines

Some medicines may interact with chemotherapy drugs. This interaction can affect both how well the chemotherapy works and the severity of side effects. The doctor should be given a list of all medicines the person is taking, including prescription medicines, herbal remedies, vitamins, and any over-the-counter medicines (such as aspirin, laxatives, cold pills, pain relievers, and so on). Include the name of each drug, the dose, how often it is taken, and the reason for taking it.

The doctor should review the list and let the person know whether any of the medicines need to be stopped before chemotherapy begins. After treatments begin, be sure to check with the doctor before the person begins taking any new medicines (apart from those in the chemotherapy regimen) or stops taking any of the medicines on the original list.

Undergoing Chemotherapy

Chemotherapy may be given at home, in a doctor's office, in a clinic, in a hospital's outpatient department, or in the hospital itself. Taking chemotherapy by mouth or by injection generally feels the same as taking other medicines by these methods. Having an IV injection usually feels like having blood drawn for a blood test. Some people feel coolness or another unusual sensation in the area of the injection when the IV is started. Report any feelings of discomfort or pain.

Many people have little or no trouble having the IV in their hand or lower arm. If a person has a hard time for any reason or if it becomes difficult to insert the needle into a vein for each treatment, it may be possible to use a catheter or port. Catheters and ports cause no pain or discomfort if they are properly placed and cared for, though the person is usually aware that they are there.

Some people are able to keep working while undergoing chemotherapy. It may be possible to schedule treatments late in the day or right before the weekend, so they interfere with work as little as possible.

Most people preparing for chemotherapy are concerned about whether they will have side effects and what the side effects may be. Side effects can vary a great deal between people, depending on the type and dosage of drugs given, the length of treatment, and how the person's body responds. The most common side effects of chemotherapy include the following:

- loss of appetite
- nausea and/or vomiting
- mouth sores
- hair loss
- fatigue (due to low red blood cell counts)
- lowered resistance to infection (due to low white blood cell counts)
- easy bruising or bleeding (due to low blood platelet counts)

In addition, each chemotherapy drug may have some of its own unique side effects. The doctor can provide information on what side effects might be expected.

Evaluating Progress

The person's health care team will likely use several methods to measure how well chemotherapy is working. People with cancer can expect to have frequent physical examinations, blood tests, and imaging tests, including CT scans, MRIs, and x-ray studies. It may take several weeks or months after starting treatment to get a feel for whether treatment is working. Do not hesitate to ask about test results and what they mean, especially in terms of progress.

Whereas tests and exams can tell a lot about how chemotherapy is working, side effects tell very little. Sometimes people think that if they do not have side effects, the drugs are not working. Side effects vary so much, however, from person to person and from drug to drug that they are not a good indication of whether the treatment is having an effect.

IV. Bone Marrow and Peripheral Blood Stem Cell Transplants

Bone marrow and peripheral blood stem cell transplants are used to treat people with cancers of the bone marrow or with certain types of cancer that require very high doses of chemotherapy and/or radiation. Chemotherapy drugs damage quickly dividing cells such as those in the bone marrow, where new blood cells are made. Even though higher doses of these drugs might be more effective in treating cancer, they are not given because the severe damage to bone marrow cells would cause lethal shortages of blood cells. A stem cell transplant allows doctors to use higher doses of chemotherapy. After treatment is finished, the person receives a transplant of blood-forming stem cells to restore the bone marrow.

The blood-forming stem cells that are used for a transplant are obtained either from the blood (for a peripheral blood stem cell transplant, or PBSCT) or from the bone marrow (for a bone marrow transplant, or BMT). Bone marrow transplants were more common in the past, but they have largely been replaced by peripheral blood stem cell transplants. Peripheral blood stem cells are obtained through a process similar to blood donation, whereas bone marrow donation is usually performed in an operating room under general anesthesia.

Destroying marrow may be a part of treatment for diseases that affect the bone marrow (such as leukemia), or destroyed marrow may simply be a side effect of treatment for cancers that affect other parts of the body. In any case, BMT and PBSCT allow stem cells that were damaged by treatment to be replaced with healthy stem cells that can make the blood cells the person needs.

Types of Stem Cell Transplants

There are two main types of stem cell transplants. They differ with regard to the source of the blood-forming stem cells.

In an *autologous stem cell transplant*, a person's own stem cells are removed from his or her bone marrow or peripheral (circulating) blood. They are collected in the weeks before treatment. The cells are frozen and stored while the person gets treatment (high-dose chemotherapy and/or radiation) and then are reinfused into the person's blood.

In an *allogeneic stem cell transplant*, the stem cells come from someone else—usually a donor whose tissue type is almost identical to the patient's. Tissue type is based on substances that are present on the surface of cells in the body. These substances can cause the immune system to react against the transplanted stem cells. Therefore, the closer the tissue match between the donor and recipient, the better the chance the transplanted cells will begin making new blood cells. The donor could be a sibling, a parent, or an unrelated donor. Stem cells from unrelated donors come from volunteers whose tissue type has been stored in a central registry and matched with that of the patient. Sometimes umbilical cord stem cells are used; these cells come from blood drained from the umbilical cord and placenta after a baby is born and the umbilical cord is cut.

With both autologous and allogeneic transplants, the blood-forming stem cells are carefully frozen and stored before the person undergoes treatment. The person then receives high-dose chemotherapy and/or whole body radiation treatment. (Radiation shields are used to protect the lungs, heart, and kidneys from damage during radiation therapy to the whole body.) This radiation destroys remaining cancer cells, but it also kills all or most healthy cells in the bone marrow. After treatment, the frozen stem cells are thawed and returned to the body as in a blood transfusion. The stem cells settle into the person's bone marrow over the next several days and start to grow and make new blood cells.

Nonmyeloablative Transplants

Standard allogeneic and autologous transplants using high-dose chemotherapy and/or radiation therapy are considered myeloablative transplants because the treatment causes extreme suppression of the bone marrow, meaning bone marrow cells are severely or completely depleted. A newer option for some people may be a nonmyeloablative transplant (also known as a mini-transplant or reduced-intensity transplant). Most people over the age of about fifty-five cannot tolerate a transplant that uses high doses of chemotherapy. In a mini-transplant, a person gets lower doses of chemotherapy and radiation, which do not completely destroy the cells in the bone marrow. The person then receives the donor stem cells or his or her own stem cells. These cells enter the body and establish a new immune system, which sees the cancer cells as foreign and attacks them.

By using small doses of certain chemotherapy drugs and low doses of total body radiation, an allogeneic transplant can still work with much less toxicity. In fact, a person can receive a non-myeloablative transplant as an outpatient procedure. Doctors are still learning about the best ways to use these transplants.

The Transplant Procedure

In the weeks before the actual transplant, the person will likely need several examinations and laboratory tests. Doctors check the person's medical condition, looking for signs of infection or damage to organs from previous treatment. A dental examination is often recommended to make sure the mouth is as healthy as possible before treatment begins because treatment will likely cause the mouth and gums to become sensitive and easily infected. If the stem cells are coming from the person with cancer, they will be taken out close to the time of reinfusion or transplant.

Usually, an IV catheter is surgically placed in one of the large veins in the chest. The catheter is used for drawing blood samples; for giving blood or blood products, medicines, and nutrition support; and for infusing the stem cells. The person getting the stem cell transplant may be admitted to the hospital or receive treatment as an outpatient, depending on a number of factors. If the transplant is performed as an inpatient procedure, the person is usually admitted to the hospital on the day before chemotherapy begins. He or she will usually stay in the hospital through chemotherapy and remain there until the newly transplanted stem cells have started to make new blood cells again. If the transplant is performed as an outpatient procedure, the person and any caregivers must watch for complications requiring the doctor's attention. Unless the person lives near the transplant center, he or she will be asked to stay in a hotel nearby.

Once the person has undergone treatment, the new stem cells are given through the IV catheter, just as in a blood transfusion. The stem cells migrate to the bone marrow. People who receive someone else's stem cells (an allogeneic transplant) are given drugs that suppress their immune system so that the new bone marrow will not be rejected or destroyed.

For the next three to four weeks, the person is given as much supportive therapy as necessary. This therapy can include IV nutrition, antibiotics to treat infections, red blood cell and/or platelet transfusions, and other medicines.

Usually around two to three weeks after the stem cells have been infused, they begin making new white blood cells. This step is followed by new platelet production and, several weeks later, by new red blood cell production. Because of the high risk of serious infections right after treatment, the person remains in protective isolation (where visitors and exposure to germs are kept to a minimum) until his or her absolute neutrophil count, or ANC, (a measure of the person's white blood cell levels) rises above five hundred. The patient can usually leave the hospital when the ANC nears one thousand.

Follow-up Care

People typically make regular visits to the outpatient transplant clinic for about six months, after which time their care is continued by their personal oncologist or internist. At this point, they only come back to the clinic for regular examinations or if they have symptoms that require attention from their doctor.

Many people need a full year to recover physically and psychologically from a transplant. Even after that period, life may not return to the way it was before the illness: medicine to prevent transplant rejection may be needed indefinitely, and the person's lifestyle may have to change to help prevent fatigue, avoid infections, and cope with the long-term effects of treatment.

Family caregivers are also affected by the long-term effort of caring for people who undergo stem cell transplant. Home health nurses can assist the family greatly during recovery.

V. Biotherapy

Biotherapy is treatment that stimulates a person's immune system to attack cancer cells. It is also known as immunotherapy, biologic therapy, or biological therapy. Biotherapy is sometimes used by itself to treat cancer, but it is most often used along with or after another type of treatment to add to its effects. It still has a fairly small role in treating most types of cancer. Its main role at this time is making other forms of treatment more effective.

The immune system is a collection of organs, special cells, and substances that help protect the body from disease. Immune system cells and the substances they make circulate through the body to protect it from germs and, to some extent, from cancer. The substances immune system cells make to communicate with each other are known as *cytokines*. Examples of cytokines include *interleukins* and *interferons*. Some of these substances cause other immune system cells to grow or become more active, improving the body's ability to fight cancer. Cytokines can play many roles in cancer treatment, including slowing or stopping tumor cell growth and acting to help healthy cells, particularly immune system cells, control cancer. Scientists have now discovered how to make some of these substances in the laboratory.

There are two main types of biotherapy. Active biotherapies stimulate the body's immune system to fight the disease. Passive biotherapies do not rely on the body to start the attack on the disease; instead, they use immune system components (such as antibodies) that are made in a laboratory. These are some of the most common types of biotherapy:

- monoclonal antibodies
- other targeted biotherapies that carry toxins to cancer cells
- cancer vaccines and other active biotherapies

Biotherapy is given in one of two ways:

- ***injection into a vein, usually on the hand or forearm.*** The drug may be given over a few minutes—called an "IV push"—or as an infusion that can last several hours.
- ***injection into a muscle, under the skin, or directly into a cancerous area in the skin.***

Most biotherapies can be given on an outpatient basis, either daily or a few times a week. Some can even be given at home, either by the person with cancer or by the caregiver. If you are helping to administer the person's treatment at home, the health care team will explain what you need to do. Before agreeing to handle this task at home, make sure you are comfortable with the procedure and that all of your questions have been answered.

Side Effects of Biotherapy

Like other forms of cancer treatment, biotherapy can have side effects. Some of the main side effects include flu-like symptoms and sleepiness. For more information on the different forms of biotherapy and their side effects, visit **cancer.org**.

VI. Targeted Therapy

As scientists have learned more about the changes in cells that cause cancer, they have been able to develop newer drugs that specifically target these changes. Targeted therapies block the growth and spread of cancer by interfering with specific molecules involved in tumor growth and progression. These targeted drugs work differently from standard chemotherapy drugs. They often have different and less severe side effects. They may be used alone or in combination with other treatments, such as chemotherapy.

Most targeted therapies are either small-molecule drugs or monoclonal antibodies. Small-molecule drugs are typically able to penetrate cells and can act on targets inside the cell. Monoclonal antibodies usually cannot get through the cell's surface and are used against targets that are on the surface of the cell or outside the cell. There a number of different targeted therapies currently in use, and the vast majority of them fall into one of these two categories.

Monoclonal antibodies are man-made versions of immune system proteins. They can be designed to attack very specific targets on cancer cells. These drugs are given by IV infusion, usually over the course of a few hours. Monoclonal antibodies can have different side effects depending on their target, but all of them have a small chance of causing an allergic reaction.

Small molecule inhibitors are chemicals designed to block the action of a specific part of a cancer cell. The possible side effects of these drugs can vary, depending on their target. The medicine is taken at home in pill form, but it is strong, so it is important for people to take it on schedule and inform the health care team if there are any problems.

Researchers are studying a number of types of targeted therapies in clinical trials, but some drugs are already in widespread use. These are some of the most common examples:

- ***Enzyme inhibitors.*** Some targeted therapies block specific enzymes that act as signals for cancer cells to grow. Enzyme inhibitors are used to treat some types of leukemia and cancers of the breast, colon, lung, head, and neck, among others. Enzyme inhibitors may help some chemotherapy drugs work better. While these drugs tend not to have the harsh side effects of chemotherapy drugs, one possible side effect is an acne-like rash on the face and chest.

- ***Angiogenesis inhibitors.*** Angiogenesis inhibitors target the new blood vessels that tumors need to grow. This type of therapy is being used to treat colorectal, lung, breast, kidney, and other cancers. Possible side effects of these drugs include high blood pressure, blood clots, and abnormal bleeding.

- ***Apoptosis-inducing drugs.*** Apoptosis-inducing drugs change proteins within the cancer cells and cause the cell to die. These drugs are currently approved for the treatment of some types of lymphoma and multiple myeloma.

Because targeted therapy includes a number of different drugs with different possible side effects, it's important that a person receiving targeted therapy be made aware of any specific side effects associated with the drug or drugs prescribed.

VII. Hormonal Therapy

Hormones are naturally occurring substances that have different effects in the body. Hormonal therapy can refer to the use of hormones or the use of other substances to *block* certain hormones, with the goal of preventing the growth, spread, or recurrence of cancer.

Steroid hormones (such as prednisone and dexamethasone) are often useful to help treat cancer or to lessen symptoms or side effects of other treatments. But most hormonal therapies used to treat cancer affect sex hormones, including estrogen, progesterone, or testosterone. For example, if laboratory tests show that a breast cancer depends on estrogen to grow, a treatment (such as tamoxifen) that prevents estrogen from reaching the cancer cells may be used to treat the cancer or help prevent recurrence. The growth of some cancers, such as breast and prostate cancer, is much more likely to be fueled by hormone levels than are some other common types of cancer, such as colorectal or lung cancer. For that reason, hormonal therapy is more likely to be useful in treating these cancers.

The goal of hormonal therapy depends on the type and extent of the cancer and on what other treatments are planned or have been given. It is sometimes used with surgery or it may be used for more advanced disease to try to slow the cancer's growth. It is important to have an idea of what the goal of hormonal therapy is before treatment is started. If the goal is unclear, ask the doctor.

Therapies that affect the body's use of androgens (male hormones) are most often used to treat prostate cancer:

- *Orchiectomy (castration)* is the surgical removal of one or both of the testicles (where most testosterone is made).
- *Luteinizing hormone–releasing hormone (LHRH) analogs and antagonists* are drugs, such as leuprolide and abarelix, that work in a complex way to lower the level of hormones such as testosterone. They are given as injections every month or every few months.
- *Antiandrogens* are drugs, such as flutamide and bicalutamide, that block the body's ability to use androgens. They are taken daily as pills.
- *Estrogens* are drugs that counteract the effects of testosterone. They are used less often than in the past because of side effects such as blood clots.

Therapies that affect the body's use of estrogen or progesterone (female hormones) are used most often to treat breast cancer, though some of them may also be helpful in the treatment of endometrial cancer and other cancers.

- *Antiestrogens* are drugs that stop estrogen from reaching cancer cells. These include medicines such as tamoxifen, toremifene, and fulvestrant. Some are taken daily as pills, whereas others are given as monthly injections.
- *Aromatase inhibitors* are drugs, including letrozole and anastrozole, that are used in post-

menopausal women to stop the body from making more estrogen. They are taken daily as pills.

- *Progestins* are progesterone-like drugs sometimes used to treat endometrial or breast cancer. Examples include medroxyprogesterone and megestrol. They are taken as pills.
- *Ovarian ablation* is a treatment that stops the ovaries' ability to make estrogen. Ablation can be done by surgical removal of the ovaries (oophorectomy), radiation of the ovaries, or with such drugs as LHRH analogs.
- *Androgens* are drugs that counteract the effects of estrogen. They are used less frequently than in the past.

The possible side effects of hormonal therapy depend on the treatment being used. Some of these drugs can cause symptoms such as hot flashes or may increase the risk of other problems, including blood clots or loss of bone density. Be sure the doctor explains the possible side effects of the prescribed drugs and what symptoms to look for.

VIII. Clinical Trials

Clinical trials are carefully controlled research studies involving people. These studies test whether a new treatment is safe and how well it works. Clinical trials have led to many advances in cancer treatment.

A clinical trial is done only when there is good reason to believe that the treatment, test, or procedure being studied may be better than the standard treatment in use. Treatments used in clinical trials are often found to have real benefits and may go on to become tomorrow's standard treatment.

People in clinical trials have a team of experts taking care of them and watching their progress very carefully. Depending on the type of clinical trial, they may receive more attention (such as having more doctor visits and laboratory tests) than they would if they were treated outside of a clinical trial.

There are some risks. No one involved in the study knows in advance whether the treatment will work or exactly what side effects will occur. That is what the study is designed to find out. While most side effects go away in time, some may be long-lasting or even life-threatening. Keep in mind, though, that even standard treatments have side effects. Depending on many factors, a person may decide to enroll in a clinical trial.

Clinical trials can focus on many things:
- new uses of drugs that are already approved by the U.S. Food and Drug Administration (FDA)
- new drugs that have not yet been approved by the FDA

- nondrug treatments (such as radiation therapy)
- medical procedures (such as types of surgery)
- herbs and vitamins
- tools to improve the ways medicines or diagnostic tests are used
- medicines or procedures to relieve symptoms or improve comfort
- combinations of treatments and procedures

Researchers conduct studies of new treatments to try to answer the following questions:
- Is the treatment helpful?
- What's the best way to give it?
- Does it work better than other treatments already available?
- What side effects does the treatment cause?
- Are there more or fewer side effects than the standard treatment used now?
- Do the benefits outweigh the side effects?
- In which people is the treatment most likely to be helpful?

There are four phases of clinical trials.

Phase I Clinical Trials

The purpose of a phase I study is to find the safest way to give a new treatment to people. The cancer care team closely watches patients for any harmful side effects.

For phase I studies, the drug has already been tested in laboratory and animal studies, but the side effects in people are not fully known. Doctors start by giving very low doses of the drug to the first group and increase the doses for later groups until side effects appear or the desired effect is seen. Doctors are hoping to help the patients in the study, but the main purpose of a phase I trial is to test the safety of the drug.

Phase I clinical trials are often done in small groups of people with different cancers that have not responded to standard treatment or that keep recurring (coming back) after treatment. If a drug is found to be reasonably safe in phase I studies, it can be tested in a phase II clinical trial.

Phase II Clinical Trials

These studies are designed to see whether the drug is effective. Patients are given the safest dose, as determined from phase I studies. They are closely watched for an effect on the cancer. The cancer care team also looks for side effects. Phase II trials are often done in larger groups of people with a specific cancer type that has not responded to standard treatment. If a drug is found to be effective in phase II studies, it can be tested in a phase III clinical trial.

Phase III Clinical Trials

Phase III studies involve large numbers of patients—most often people who have just received a diagnosis for a specific type of cancer. Phase III clinical trials may enroll thousands of patients. Often, these studies are randomized, which means that patients are randomly put in one of two (or more) groups. One group (called the control group) gets the standard, most accepted treatment. The other group(s) gets the new treatment(s) being studied. All patients in phase III studies are closely watched. The study will be stopped early if many patients have side effects from the new treatment that are too severe or if one group has much better results than the others. Phase III clinical trials are needed before the FDA will approve a treatment for use by the general public.

Phase IV Clinical Trials

Once a drug has been approved by the FDA and is available for all people, it is still studied in other clinical trials (sometimes referred to as phase IV studies). This way, more can be learned about short-term and long-term side effects and safety as the drug is used in larger numbers of people with many types of diseases. Doctors can also learn more about how well the drug works and whether it might be helpful when used in other ways (such as in combination with other treatments).

Deciding to Enter a Clinical Trial

If the person with cancer would like to take part in a clinical trial, he or she should begin by asking the doctor if the clinic or hospital conducts clinical trials. All clinical trials will have certain requirements. But the decision to enroll in a clinical trial is completely up to the person. The doctors and nurses conducting the study will explain the study in detail. They will go over the possible risks and benefits and have the person read and sign an informed consent form indicating he or she understands the clinical trial and wants to take part in it. Even after the clinical trial begins, the person is free to leave the study at any time, for any reason. Taking part in a clinical trial does not keep the person from getting any other needed medical care.

To find out more about clinical trials, talk to the cancer care team. Here are some questions to ask:

- Is there a clinical trial that I should take part in?
- What is the purpose of the study?
- How might this study be of benefit to me?
- What is likely to happen in my case with, or without, this new treatment?
- What kinds of tests and treatments does the study involve?

- What does this treatment do? Has it been used before?
- Will I know which treatment I receive?
- What are my other choices and their pros and cons?
- How could the study affect my daily life?
- What side effects can I expect from the study? Can the side effects be controlled?
- Will I have to stay in the hospital? If so, how often and for how long?
- Will the study cost me anything? Will any of the treatment be free?
- If I am harmed as a result of the research, what treatment would I be entitled to?
- What type of long-term follow-up care is part of the study?
- Has the treatment been used to treat other types of cancer?

Finding Out More About Clinical Trials

The American Cancer Society offers a clinical trials matching service for use by patients, their family, or friends. You can reach this service at **800-303-5691** or **http://clinicaltrials.cancer.org**.

Based on the information you give about your cancer type, stage, and previous treatments, this service can put together a list of clinical trials that match your medical needs. The service will also ask where you live and whether you are willing to travel so that it can look for a treatment center that you can get to. You can also get a list of current clinical trials by calling the National Cancer Institute's Cancer Information Service toll-free at **800-4-CANCER (800-422-6237)** or by visiting the NCI clinical trials Web site at **www.cancer.gov/clinicaltrials**.

APPENDIX B

Food Safety Guidelines for People Undergoing Cancer Treatment*

When a person's immune system is weakened, the first step in staying free from infection is being aware of the bacteria and other organisms that could cause an illness and avoiding or getting rid of them. The choices you make when buying and handling foods, preparing meals, and dining out can affect exposure to infectious organisms. Following food safety guidelines reduces the risk of infection.

Food Safety at Home

The following food safety guidelines are adapted from guidelines created by the Seattle Cancer Care Alliance for people with weakened immune systems. Talk to your doctor about whether you should follow these guidelines during your treatment.

Personal Hygiene
- Wash hands frequently—before and after each step of food preparation—with plenty of soap and hot, running water for at least twenty seconds.
- Wash hands before eating and after using the restroom, handling garbage, answering the phone, or touching pets.

Preparing Foods
- Use different knives and cutting boards for meat, produce, and bread.
- Do not taste food with the same utensil used for stirring.
- Wash fruits and vegetables thoroughly under cold running water just before use and scrub lightly with a vegetable brush to remove dirt and debris.
- Individually rinse the leaves of leafy vegetables such as lettuce or cabbage. Wash all packaged salads and other prepared produce under cold running water, even when they are marked as prewashed.

*Adapted from *American Cancer Society Complete Guide to Nutrition for Cancer Survivors: Eating Well, Staying Well During and After Cancer*. 2nd ed. (Atlanta, GA: American Cancer Society, 2010).

- Keep track of the "use by" dates on packaged and prepared produce and do not eat items that are expired.
- Wash and softly scrub with a vegetable brush the outside of all fruits and vegetables (such as oranges, melons, and bananas), even if the produce will be peeled or cut. This will prevent any bacteria or debris on the outside of the fruit from being transferred to the fruit itself.
- Wash the tops of canned foods before opening, and clean the can opener after each use.

Thawing and Cooking Foods

- Cook eggs until the yolks and whites are firm. Cook egg dishes, custards, egg sauces, and casseroles that include eggs to a minimum internal temperature of 160°F, using a cooking thermometer as a guide.
- Cook meats until they are no longer pink and the juices run clear. The only way you can be sure that meat has been cooked to a safe temperature is by using a food thermometer and following the recommended minimum cooking temperatures specified in the table on page 292.
- Heat any leftovers to 165°F, using a cooking thermometer as a guide.
- Thaw meat, fish, or poultry in the refrigerator away from raw fruits and vegetables and other prepared foods. Place on a dish to catch drips. Cook defrosted meat right away, and do not refreeze without cooking it thoroughly first. If you are in a hurry, you may thaw meat in the microwave, but cook it immediately after thawing.
- When microwaving, rotate the dish a quarter turn once or twice during cooking if there is no turntable in the microwave oven. This prevents cold spots in food where bacteria can survive.
- Use a lid or vented plastic wrap to thoroughly heat leftovers in the microwave. Stir several times during reheating. When food is heated thoroughly (to a minimum of 165°F, using a cooking thermometer as a guide), cover and let sit two minutes before serving.
- Cut tofu into half-inch cubes and boil for five minutes before using. (This process is not necessary if you are using tofu in shelf-stable packaging for which refrigeration is not needed until the product is opened.)

Refrigerating and Storing Foods

- Purchase and use a refrigerator thermometer (available at many grocery and hardware stores). After foods are prepared and/or heated to their recommended temperatures, hold foods at safe temperatures: cold food below 40°F and hot foods above 165°F, using a cooking thermometer as a guide.

- Never leave perishable food out of the refrigerator for more than two hours; throw away food left out longer than two hours.
- Never re-refrigerate or re-freeze leftovers not eaten within the food storage limits on page 293. Throw it out!
- Refrigerate fruits and vegetables. Discard fruits and vegetables that are slimy, mushy, or show mold.
- Throw out foods that look or smell strange. Never taste them! When in doubt—throw it out!

Drinking Water

- Do not drink well water unless it is tested yearly for coliform bacteria.
- Do not drink water straight from lakes, rivers, streams, or springs.
- If using a water service other than the local city water service, drink bottled or distilled water.
- If using a home water-filtering system with city water, change the water filter regularly according to the manufacturer's instructions.
- When in doubt about your water's safety, simply bring the water to a rolling boil for one minute. After boiling, store the water in a clean covered container in the refrigerator, and throw out any unused water after seventy-two hours.

Work Surfaces and Kitchen Equipment

- Use separate cutting boards for cooked foods and raw foods. Cut on plastic or glass cutting boards when cutting raw meat and poultry. Wooden boards used exclusively for raw meat and poultry are acceptable, but use a different board for cutting other foods, such as produce or bread.
- Wash cutting boards after each use in hot, soapy water; rinse and air dry or pat dry with fresh paper towels. Nonporous acrylic, plastic, glass, and solid-wood boards can be washed in the dishwasher (laminated boards may crack and split).
- Make up a sanitizing solution for general use on kitchen work surfaces, cutting boards, and other utensils. Mix two teaspoons of household bleach in one quart of water. After using the sanitizing solution, rinse with clean water, wipe with a paper towel, and allow to air dry. Alternatively, use a commercial sanitizing agent and follow the directions on the product.
- Clean food particles off of the microwave oven, toaster, can opener, and blender and mixer blades. Remove blender blades and the bottom ring when washing the blender container. Use a bleach solution of two tablespoons of household bleach to one quart of water to sanitize these items.

- Keep the counter and kitchen surfaces free of food particles. Clean regularly with a bleach solution.

Sink Area

- Keep soap available for hand washing.
- Use paper towels for drying hands.
- Replace dishcloths and dishtowels daily.
- Replace sponges at least weekly.
- Sanitize sponges daily in a solution of two tablespoons of household bleach and one quart of water or place in dishwasher. Or use paper towels instead of sponges while your immune system may be compromised.
- Do not store food supplies under the kitchen sink. Do not store chemicals and cleaning solutions near or over food supplies.
- Use liquid dish soap when hand washing dishes, pans, and utensils.
- Air dry dishes instead of towel-drying them.

Refrigerator and Freezer

- Keep the refrigerator clean: clean up spills immediately, discard food scraps, and sanitize shelves and doors regularly with a solution of two tablespoons of household bleach to one quart of water.
- Keep the refrigerator temperature between 34°F and 40°F.
- Keep the freezer temperature below 2°F.
- Cool hot foods, uncovered, in the refrigerator in shallow containers; cover storage containers tightly after cooling. Freeze what you do not plan to use within the next two to three days.
- Throw away all refrigerated, cooked leftovers after three days (date foods to keep track of the age of leftovers).
- Throw out eggs with cracked shells or eggs with chicken feces on them.
- Throw out foods older than their "use by" expiration dates.
- Throw out entire food packages or containers with any mold present, including yogurt, cheese, cottage cheese, fruit, vegetables, jelly, and bread and pastry products.
- Throw out freezer-burned foods.

Cupboards and Pantry

- Throw out—without tasting or opening—any can with a bulge, leak, crack, or deep indentation in the seam area.

- Rotate food stock so older items are used first. Do not use foods older than their "use by" dates.
- Keep food storage areas clean, and monitor for signs of insect or rodent contamination.
- Review the processing used in preparing home-canned foods to be sure it is appropriate for the acidity of the food, size of the container, and elevation above sea level. Look for mold and leaks. Check seals. If you suspect a home-canned food may not have been processed properly (for example, if the lid bulges, or if the food has any bad odor or unusual characteristics after opening), throw it away. Use home-canned foods within one year of canning, as chemical changes may occur.

Food Safety Outside the Home

It is easier to control bacteria and other organisms in your home than in other environments. But you can keep an eye on food safety when you are outside the home by following these tips:

Grocery Shopping

- Wipe down the handle of the grocery cart or basket with a sanitary wipe (usually available at the entrance of grocery stores).
- Shop for shelf-stable items first, such as canned and boxed foods. Select frozen and refrigerated foods last, especially during summer months.
- Check "sell by" and "use by" dates on dairy products, eggs, cereals, canned foods, and other goods. Purchase only the freshest products.
- Check the packaging and "use by" dates on fresh meats, poultry, and seafood. Do not purchase any products that are out of date.
- Reject damaged, swollen, rusted, or deeply dented cans. Make sure that packaged and boxed foods are properly sealed.
- Select unblemished fruits and vegetables that look and smell fresh. Avoid wilted produce.
- Avoid delicatessen foods.
- In the bakery, avoid unrefrigerated cream- and custard-containing desserts and pastries.
- Avoid foods from self-serve or bulk containers.
- Resist trying free food samples.
- Open egg cartons to be sure you do not buy cracked eggs.
- Do not buy unrefrigerated eggs.
- Ask that meat, poultry, and fish be placed in separate bags from fresh produce at the checkout.

- Use a "stay-cool" bag to transport refrigerated or frozen products for the trip home from the grocery store.
- Refrigerate or freeze perishables promptly, and never leave perishables in a hot car.

Dining Out

- Eat early to avoid crowds.
- Ask that fresh food be prepared in fast-food restaurants.
- Ask whether fruit juices are pasteurized, and do not drink nonpasteurized juice.
- Avoid raw prepared fruits and vegetables; eat these items at home where you can clean them thoroughly.
- Request single-serving condiment packages, and avoid self-serve bulk condiment containers. Do not eat salsa or other condiments that are unrefrigerated and used by multiple people at a restaurant.
- Avoid salad bars, delicatessens, buffets, smorgasbords, potlucks, and sidewalk vendors. These are high-risk food sources because of potentially improper food storage or holding temperatures and poor hygiene by those handling the food.
- Consider the general condition of the restaurant before eating there. Are the plates, glasses, and utensils clean? Are the restrooms clean and stocked with soap and paper towels? The cleanliness of the restaurant itself may indicate the cleanliness and care involved in food preparation.
- Avoid soft-serve ice cream, milk shakes, and frozen yogurt dispensed from a machine. Avoid self-serve ice cream and self-serve beverage and ice machines.

Nutrition Suggestions for People with Weakened Immune Systems

There are certain foods that all people should avoid, regardless of the state of their immune systems. These foods can harbor high levels of bacteria, and eating them can lead to contracting a foodborne illness:

- Uncooked vegetable sprouts (all types, including alfalfa, radish, broccoli, mung bean, etc.), because of a high risk of contamination with salmonella and E. coli.
- Raw or runny eggs, including nonpasteurized eggnog, uncooked Caesar salad dressing, and unbaked meringues. To avoid bacterial contamination, substitute frozen pasteurized eggs or powdered egg whites for raw eggs in recipes for uncooked foods.
- Nonpasteurized fruit and vegetable juice, unless prepared at home with washed produce.
- Undercooked meat or poultry, especially ground meats.

Within seven to fourteen days after chemotherapy, white blood counts can drop to a dangerous level. During this time, the person may be at a higher risk for infection and may need to avoid foods that are likely to harbor high levels of bacteria, including unwashed fruits or vegetables, nonpasteurized juices, and raw or undercooked fish, meats, and eggs.

If the person is neutropenic (meaning the neutrophil count is low and the person is more susceptible to infection), consider avoiding the foods listed below:

- raw or undercooked tofu
- raw or undercooked animal products, including meat, pork, game, poultry, eggs, hot dogs, luncheon meats, deli meats, sausage, and bacon
- uncooked foods containing raw eggs, such as hollandaise sauce, raw cookie dough, or homemade mayonnaise. (Liquid pasteurized egg product may be used in recipes that call for raw eggs.)
- raw or lightly cooked fish, shellfish, lox, sushi, or sashimi
- nonpasteurized milk and dairy products. (You may eat products made from pasteurized milk, including grade A milk, hard cheeses, processed cheeses, cream cheese, cottage cheese, and yogurt.)
- soft cheeses such as feta, Brie, Camembert, blue-veined (Roquefort, Stilton, Gorgonzola, and blue), or Mexican-style (such as queso blanco fresco)
- salad dressings and salsas that are not shelf-stable. (Shelf-stable refers to unopened canned, bottled, or packaged food products that can be stored at room temperature before opening; the container may require refrigeration after opening.)
- unwashed raw vegetables and fruits and those with visible mold
- raw honey. (Instead, select commercial grade A or heat-treated honey.)
- unprocessed or raw peanut butter or other nut butters
- sun tea, meaning tea that is left to steep in sunlight. (Instead, make tea with boiling water, using commercially packaged teabags.)
- nonpasteurized beer
- uncooked brewer's yeast
- untested well water

Recommended Minimum Cooking Temperatures for Eggs, Meats, Poultry, and Seafood

	PRODUCT	COOKING TEMPERATURE
Eggs, egg dishes, and casseroles	Eggs	Cook until yolks and whites are firm
	Casseroles, egg dishes, custards, egg sauces	160°F
Beef, pork, veal, lamb, rabbit, goat, game	Whole pieces of meat, chops, ribs	160°F
	Ground beef, pork, veal, lamb, rabbit, goat, game	160°F
Poultry (chicken, turkey, duck, goose)	Chicken and turkey: whole bird and dark meat (thigh, wing)	180°F
	Breast	170°F
	Ground chicken, turkey	165°F
	Stuffing (always cook in separate container outside of bird)	165°F
Ham	Fresh (raw) or precooked (to reheat)	160°F
Seafood	Fin fish (such as salmon, cod, halibut, snapper, sole, bass, trout)	Cook until opaque and flakes easily with a fork
	Shrimp, lobster, crab	Should turn red and flesh should become pearly opaque
	Scallops	Should turn milk white or opaque and firm
	Clams, mussels, oysters	Cook until shells open (may be high-risk for people with low white blood cell count or immunosuppression)
Ready-to-eat meats	Hot dogs, luncheon meats, cold cuts, deli-style meats*	Heat thoroughly until steaming

* Keep your intake of processed meats to a minimum, if they are eaten at all. Choose more nutritious, leaner meats whenever possible.

Limits for Food Storage		
	REFRIGERATOR **34–40°F**	**FREEZER** **BELOW 0–2°F**
Red meats—cooked	3 days	2 to 3 months
Red meats—raw	3 days	4 to 12 months
Poultry—cooked	3 days	4 months
Poultry—raw	1 to 2 days	9 to 12 months
Casseroles	3 days	2 to 3 months
Frozen dinners	3 days	3 to 4 months

For more information about food safety and cancer treatment, call your American Cancer Society at **800-227-2345** or visit the Web site, **cancer.org**.

REFERENCES

American Cancer Society. *Cancer Caregiving A to Z: An At-Home Guide for Patients and Families*. Atlanta, GA: American Cancer Society; 2008.

Be your own health advocate: change from passive patient to an active advocate for your own health care. WebMD Web site. http://www.webmd.com/healthy-aging/guide/be-your-own-health-advocate. Accessed September 14, 2010.

Biological therapy. National Cancer Institute Web site. http://www.cancer.gov/cancertopics/treatment/biological therapy. Updated December 29, 2004. Accessed September 14, 2010.

Blum S. *Caregiving for Your Loved One with Cancer* [booklet]. New York, NY: Cancer Care; 2008.

Caregiving: caring for a loved one with cancer—and yourself. American Cancer Society Web site. http://www.cancer.org/acs/groups/cid/documents/webcontent/003199-pdf.pdf. Updated April 26, 2010. Accessed September 13, 2010.

Caring for the patient with cancer at home: prostheses. American Cancer Society Web site. http://www.cancer.org/Treatment/TreatmentsandSideEffects/PhysicalSideEffects/DealingwithSymptomsatHome/caring-for-the-patient-with-cancer-at-home-prostheses. Updated November 12, 2009. Accessed September 14, 2010.

Clancy CM. Keeping track of your health information. Agency for Healthcare Research and Quality Web site. http://www.ahrq.gov/consumer/cc/cc061609.htm. Posted June 16, 2009. Accessed August 12, 2010.

Clancy CM. Why it's wise to use a health advocate. Agency for Healthcare Research and Quality Web site. http://www.ahrq.gov/consumer/cc/cc070610.htm. Posted July 6, 2010. Accessed August 12, 2010.

Fact sheet: biological therapies for cancer: questions and answers. National Cancer Institute Web site. http://www.cancer.gov/cancertopics/factsheet/Therapy/biological. Updated June 13, 2006. Accessed September 14, 2010.

Fact sheet: targeted cancer therapies. National Cancer Institute Web site. http://www.cancer.gov/cancertopics/factsheet/Therapy/targeted. Updated June 21, 2010. Accessed September 14, 2010.

Fernald CD, Cook JR, Gutman CA; Family Caregiver Project, University of North Carolina, Charlotte. Caring Families. Rockville, MD: U.S. Department of Health and Human Services.

Financial help for people with cancer. CancerCare Web Site. http://www.cancercare.org/pdf/fact_sheets/fs_financial_en.pdf. Accessed March 10, 2010.

First aid for seizures. Epilepsy Foundation Web site. http://www.epilepsyfoundation.org/about/firstaid/. Accessed August 26, 2010.

Grant BL, Bloch AS, Hamilton KK, Thomson CA. *American Cancer Society Complete Guide to Nutrition for Cancer Survivors: Eating Well, Staying Well During and After Cancer*. 2nd ed. Atlanta, GA: American Cancer Society; 2010.

Hand-foot syndrome (HFS) or Palmar-Plantar Erythrodysesthesia (PPE). Breastcancer.org Web site. http://www.breastcancer.org/treatment/side_effects/hand_foot_synd.jsp. Updated July 30, 2008. Accessed November 8, 2010.

Health insurance and financial assistance for the cancer patient. American Cancer Society Web site. http://www.cancer.org/docroot/MLT/content/MLT_1x_Medical_Insurance_and_Financial_Assistance_for_the_ Cancer_Patient.asp. Updated June 8, 2009. Accessed March 1, 2010.

Health Outlook. How to be your own health advocate. Health Outlook Web site, http://www.health-outlook.com/?p=258. Posted January 17, 2009. Accessed August 12, 2010.

Hermann JF, Wojtkowiak SL, Houts PS, Kahn SB. *Helping People Cope: A Guide for Families Facing Cancer.* Harrisburg, PA: Pennsylvania Department of Health; 2001.

Houts PS, ed. *American College of Physicians Home Care Guide for Advanced Cancer.* Philadelphia, PA: American College of Physicians; 1997.

Houts PS, ed. *Eldercare at Home.* 2nd ed. New York, NY: American Geriatric Society Foundation for Health in Aging; 2004.

Lymphedema (PDQ®). National Cancer Institute Web site. http://www.cancer.gov/cancertopics/pdq/ supportivecare/lymphedema/patient/allpages. Accessed September 14, 2010.

Lymphedema: what every woman with breast cancer should know. American Cancer Society Web site. http://www.cancer.org/Treatment/TreatmentsandSideEffects/PhysicalSideEffects/Lymphedema/WhatEveryWoman withBreastCancerShouldKnow/index. Updated March 5, 2009. Accessed September 14, 2010.

Mattern AL. Be your own health advocate. EmpowHer Web site. http://www.empowher.com/wellness/content/ be-your-own-health-advocate. Accessed August 12, 2010.

Murphy DP, Cleveland MJ. Transitional care: how to minimize errors and maximize outcomes. Cancer Network Web site. http://www.cancernetwork.com/print/article/10162/40649. Posted November 1, 2006. Accessed September 8, 2010.

National Endowment for Financial Education. In treatment: financial guidance for cancer survivors and their families. American Cancer Society Web site. http://www.cancer.org/acs/groups/content/@healthpromotions/ documents/document/acsq-020182.pdf. Posted August 2009. Accessed September 16, 2010.

Nearing the end of life. American Cancer Society Web site. http://www.cancer.org/Treatment/NearingtheEndofLife/ NearingtheEndofLife/index. Updated May 6, 2009. Accessed September 13, 2010.

Nosebleeds: first aid. Mayo Clinic Web site. http://www.mayoclinic.com/health/first-aid-nosebleeds/HQ00105. Updated December 11, 2009. Accessed September 13, 2010.

Patient's bill of rights. American Cancer Society Web site. http://www.cancer.org/Treatment/FindingandPaying forTreatment/UnderstandingFinancialandLegalMatters/patients-bill-of-rights. Accessed August 12, 2010.

Rush University Medical Center. Helping older adults transition from hospital to home. Medical News Today Web site. http://www.medicalnewstoday.com/articles/158996.php. Posted July 28, 2009. Accessed September 15, 2010.

Singer A. Improving the transition from hospital to home. Health Leaders Media Web site. http://www.healthleadersmedia.com/content/215315/topic/WS_HLM2_QUA/Improving-the-transition-from-hospital-to-home.html. Posted July 17, 2008. Accessed September 15, 2010.

Skin changes caused by targeted therapies. American Cancer Society Web site. http://www.cancer.org/Treatment/TreatmentsandSideEffects/PhysicalSideEffects/ChemotherapyEffects/skin-changes-caused-by-targeted-therapies. Accessed November 8, 2010.

Sources of financial assistance. CancerCare Web Site. http://www.cancercare.org/pdf/fact_sheets/fs_Financial_Sources.pdf. Accessed March 10, 2010.

Stomas (or ostomies). American Cancer Society Web site. http://www.cancer.org/Treatment/TreatmentsandSideEffects/PhysicalSideEffects/DealingwithSymptomsatHome/caring-for-the-patient-with-cancer-at-home-stomas-or-ostomies. Updated November 12, 2009. Accessed September 14, 2010.

Transitional care planning (PDQ®). National Cancer Institute Web site. http://www.cancer.gov/cancertopics/pdq/supportivecare/transitionalcare/Patient. Updated August 31, 2010. Accessed September 13, 2010.

Vachani CV. Patient guide to hand-foot syndrome. OncoLink Web site. http://www.oncolink.org/treatment/article.cfm?c=2&s=13&id=384. Accessed November 8, 2010.

When someone you love has advanced cancer. http://www.cancer.gov/cancertopics/coping/when-someone-you-love-has-advanced-cancer. National Cancer Institute Web site. Updated July 2009. Posted September 2009. Accessed September 16, 2010.

When someone you love is being treated for cancer. National Cancer Institute Web site. http://www.cancer.gov/cancertopics/coping/when-someone-you-love-is-treated. Posted September 2005. Accessed September 16, 2010.

When your parent has cancer: a guide for teens. National Cancer Institute Web site. http://www.cancer.gov/cancertopics/coping/when-your-parent-has-cancer. Posted September 2005. Accessed September 16, 2010.

RESOURCE GUIDE

American Cancer Society

250 Williams Street
Atlanta, GA 30303-1002
Toll-free: 800-227-2345
Internet: www.cancer.org

The American Cancer Society is the nationwide community-based voluntary health organization dedicated to eliminating cancer as a major health problem by preventing cancer, saving lives, and diminishing suffering from cancer through research, education, advocacy, and service. Headquartered in Atlanta, Georgia, the American Cancer Society provides educational materials, information, and patient services. A comprehensive resource for all your cancer-related questions, the Society can also put you in touch with community resources in your area. See page 317 for information on support programs and services.

General Cancer Resources

Cancer Care, Inc.

275 Seventh Avenue, 22nd Floor
New York, NY 10001
Cancer Care Counseling Toll-free Line: 800-813-HOPE (800-813-4673)
Telephone: 212-712-8400
Fax: 212-719-0263
E-mail: info@cancercare.org
Internet: www.cancercare.org

Cancer Care is a nonprofit social service agency that provides counseling and guidance to help cancer patients, their families and friends cope with the impact of cancer. Cancer Care offers support groups; teleconferences for patients, friends, and family members; workshops, seminars and clinics; a newsletter and other publications. Cancer Care also provides a financial assistance program for constituents in New Jersey, New York, and Connecticut. The Cancer Care Web site has detailed information on cancer, cancer treatment, clinical trials, services, and links to other cancer-related sites.

National Cancer Institute

6116 Executive Boulevard, Room 3036A
Bethesda, MD 20892-8322
Cancer Information Toll-free Line: 800-4CANCER (800-422-6237)
Telephone: 301-496-5583
TTY: 800-332-8615
Cancer Fax Service: 301-402-5874
Internet: www.cancer.gov

The National Cancer Institute (NCI) provides information on cancer research, diagnosis, and treatment to patients and health care providers. Callers are automatically connected to the office serving their region. The service offers free publications and the opportunity to speak directly with a cancer specialist who is trained to provide accurate information on treatment and prevention of cancer and to make appropriate referrals.

National Coalition for Cancer Survivorship

1010 Wayne Avenue, Suite 770
Silver Spring, MD 20910
Toll-free: 888-650-9127
Telephone: 301-650-9127
Fax: 301-565-9670
E-mail: info@canceradvocacy.org
Internet: www.canceradvocacy.org

The National Coalition for Cancer Survivorship (NCCS) is a network of independent organizations working in the area of cancer survivorship and support. Its primary goal is to generate a nationwide awareness of cancer survivorship. NCCS serves as an information clearinghouse and as an advocacy group.

American Psychosocial Oncology Society

154 Hansen Road, Suite 201
Charlottesville, VA 22911
Toll-free: 866-276-7443
Telephone: 434-293-5350
Fax: 434-977-1856
Internet: http://www.apos-society.org

American Psychosocial Oncology Society (APOS) explores innovative methods to enhance the recognition and treatment of psychological, social, behavioral, and spiritual aspects of cancer. They provide clinical information, education, and a hotline for counseling and support services in order to promote the well-being of patients with cancer and families at all stages of disease. They also strive to raise the level of awareness of health professionals and the public about psychological, social, behavioral, and spiritual domains of care for patients with cancer.

American Society of Clinical Oncology

2318 Mill Road, Suite 800
Alexandria, VA 22314
Toll-free: 888-282-2552
Telephone: 571-483-1300
E-mail: membermail@asco.org
Internet: www.asco.org
CancerNet: www.peoplelivingwithcancer.org

The American Society of Clinical Oncology (ASCO) has information about cancer doctors, research, treatment, and patient care. The ASCO-sponsored *CancerNet* Web site provides information on types of cancer, coping, and patient support organizations.

Association of Oncology Social Work

100 North 20th Street, 4th Floor
Philadelphia, PA 19103
Phone: 215-599-6093
Fax: 215-564-2175
E-mail: info@aosw.org
Internet: www.aosw.org

Oncology social work is the primary professional discipline that provides psychosocial services to cancer patients, their families, and caregivers. Oncology social workers connect patients and their families with community, state, national, and international resources. The Association of Oncology Social Work (AOSW) and its members work to increase awareness about the social, emotional, educational, and spiritual needs of cancer patients through research, writing, workshops and lectures, and collaborations with other patient advocacy groups and national and international oncology organizations whose primary focus is access to quality care for cancer patients.

Oncology Nursing Society

125 Enterprise Drive
Pittsburgh, PA 15275
Toll-free: 866-257-4ONS
Telephone: 412-859-6100
Fax: 877-369-5497
E-mail: customer.service@ons.org
Internet: www.ons.org

The Oncology Nursing Society (ONS) is a professional organization of more than thirty thousand registered nurses and other health care providers dedicated to excellence in patient care, education, research, and administration in oncology nursing. The overall mission of ONS is to promote excellence in oncology nursing and quality cancer care.

The Wellness Community

919 Eighteenth Street, NW
Washington, DC 20006
Telephone: 202-659-9709
Fax: 202-659-9703
Internet: www.thewellnesscommunity.org

The Wellness Community (TWC) is an international nonprofit organization dedicated to providing support, education and hope to people with cancer and their loved ones. Through participation in support groups, educational workshops, nutrition and exercise programs, and stress-reduction classes, people affected by cancer learn vital skills that enable them to regain control, reduce isolation, and restore hope, regardless of the stage of their disease. Most importantly, TWC provides a home-like setting where people affected by cancer can connect with and learn from others. All TWC programs are free of charge. There are more than one hundred locations worldwide.

Caregiver Resources

The Center for Family Caregivers

Tad Publishing Company
P.O. Box 224
Park Ridge, IL 60068
Telephone: 773-343-6341
Internet: www.caregiving.com

The Center for Family Caregivers is a grassroots organization provides practical information on being a caregiver, managing the stress of caregiving, and solutions for caregiving situations.

Family Caregiver Alliance

180 Montgomery Street, Suite 1100
San Francisco, CA 94104
Toll-free: 800-445-8106
Telephone: 415-434-3388
E-mail: info@caregiver.org
Internet: www.caregiver.org

The Family Caregiver Alliance (FCA) is a nonprofit organization designed to address the needs of families and friends providing long-term care at home. FCA offers programs at the national, state, and local level to support and sustain caregivers. The Web site contains fact sheets, online support groups, newsletters, and links to other resources.

National Alliance for Caregiving

4720 Montgomery Lane, 5th Floor
Bethesda, MD 20814
E-mail: info@caregiving.org
Internet: www.caregiving.org

The National Alliance for Caregiving is a nonprofit coalition of national organizations focusing on issues of family caregiving. Alliance members include grassroots organizations, professional associations, service organizations, disease-specific organizations, a government agency, and corporations. The Alliance was created to conduct research, do policy analysis, develop national programs, increase public awareness of family caregiving issues, work to strengthen state and local caregiving coalitions, and represent the U.S. caregiving community internationally. Recognizing that family caregivers provide important societal and financial contributions toward maintaining the well-being of those they care for, the Alliance's mission is to be the objective national resource on family caregiving with the goal of improving the quality of life for families and care recipients.

National Association for Home Care & Hospice

228 Seventh Street, SE
Washington, DC 20003
Telephone: 202-547-7424
Fax: 202-547-3540

E-mail: hospice@nahc.org
Internet: www.nahc.org

The National Association for Home Care & Hospice (NAHC) is a professional association representing the interests of Americans who need home care (including acute, long-term, and terminal care) and the caregivers that provide them with in-home health and supportive services. Its top priorities include helping people who depend on home care by protecting Medicare and Medicaid and other government programs from erosion; moving to expand these programs and private health insurance to provide greater coverage, including assistance with long-term care; helping to increase the numbers and the qualifications of people seeking employment in the home care field; and to support and inspire those who are currently in the field. The NAHC provides a service locator and information on how to choose a home care provider.

National Family Caregivers Association

10400 Connecticut Avenue, Suite 500
Kensington, MD 20895-3944
Toll-free: 800-896-3650
Telephone: 301-942-6430
Fax: 301-942-2302
E-mail: info@thefamilycaregiver.org
Internet: http://www.nfcacares.org

The National Family Caregivers Association (NFCA) educates, supports, empowers, and speaks up for the more than fifty million Americans who care for loved ones with a chronic illness or disability or the frailties of old age. NFCA reaches across the boundaries of diagnoses, relationships, and life stages to help transform family caregivers' lives by removing barriers to health and well-being. It provides information, education, public awareness, and advocacy.

National Respite Locator Service

ARCH National Resource Center
Chapel Hill Training-Outreach Project
800 Eastowne Drive, Suite 105
Chapel Hill, NC 27514
Toll-free: 800-7-RELIEF (800-773-5433)
Internet: http://chtop.org/ARCH/National-Respite-Locator.html

Respite is a break for caregivers and families that provides temporary care to people with chronic or terminal illnesses or disabilities. Depending on the needs of a family and the resources, respite can be provided in or out of the home environment. The National Respite Locator Service helps parents, caregivers, and professionals find respite services in their state and local area.

The Rosalynn Institute for Caregiving

800 GSW Drive
Georgia Southwestern State University
Americus, GA 31709
Telephone: 229-928-1234
Fax: 229-931-2663
Internet: www.rosalynncarter.org

The Rosalynn Carter Institute establishes local, state and national partnerships committed to building quality long-term, home and community- based services. It works to provide caregivers with effective supports and make investments that promote caregiver health, skills, and resilience. Its focus includes supporting individuals and caregivers coping with chronic illness and disability.

Well Spouse Association

63 West Main Street, Suite H
Freehold, NJ 07728
Telephone: 732-577-8899
Fax: 732-577-8644
E-mail: info@wellspouse.org
Internet: www.wellspouse.org

The Well Spouse Association is a national nonprofit membership organization that advocates for and addresses the needs of individuals caring for chronically ill and/or disabled spouses/partners. They offer peer-to-peer support and educate health care professionals and the general public about the special challenges and unique issues "well" spouses face every day. They offer letter writing support groups, a bimonthly newsletter, annual conferences, weekend meetings, and referrals to local support groups throughout the country. They are also involved with other groups in educating health care professionals, politicians, and the public about the needs of "well" spouses and the importance of long-term care.

AARP

601 E Street NW
Washington, DC 20049
Toll-free: 888-OUR-AARP (888-687-2277)
Telephone: 877-627-3350
Internet: www.aarp.org.

The AARP is a membership organization that is committed to providing older adults with information on health care treatment, home care, caregiving, managed care, assisted living, insurance benefits, and resources. AARP's mission is to enhance the quality of life for all as we age, to lead positive social change, and to deliver value to members through information, advocacy, and service. They provide community service, publications, education, and advocacy. Membership is open to anyone fifty years of age or older.

U.S. Department of Health and Human Services

200 Independence Avenue, SW
Washington, DC 20201
Toll-free: 877-696-6775
Telephone: 202-619-0257

National Health Information Center (NHIC)

P. O. Box 1133
Washington, DC 20013-1133
Internet: www.health.gov and www.healthfinder.gov

The National Health Information Center (NHIC) is a health information referral service. NHIC puts health professionals and consumers who have health questions in touch with those organizations that are best able to provide answers. NHIC was established by the U.S. Department of Health and Human Services to provide key support for the healthfinder.gov Web site, a gateway to reliable consumer health information. NHIC maintains a database, accessible by Internet or telephone, with information on over eleven hundred health-related organizations and government offices that provide health information upon request.

Visiting Nurse Associations of America

900 19th Street NW, Suite 200
Washington, DC 20006
Telephone: 202-384-1420

Fax: 202-384-1444
E-mail: vnaa@vnaa.org
Internet: www.vnaa.org

The Visiting Nurse Associations of America (VNAA) is the national association of nonprofit Visiting Nurse Agencies (VNAs) and home health care providers who care for and treat approximately four million patients annually. Their mission is to support, promote, and advance the nation's network of VNAs who provide cost-effective and compassionate home health care to some of the nation's most vulnerable individuals, particularly the elderly and individuals with disabilities. Their services include advocacy, education and collaboration. They also provide members with products, resources and the support they need to accomplish their nonprofit goals. VNAs represent the largest network of nonprofit providers of influenza vaccine—over one and a half million flu shots per year. VNAA works hard to educate, advocate, and collaborate on issues facing home health care.

U.S. Administration on Aging

One Massachusetts Avenue NW
Washington, DC 20001
Telephone: 202-619-0724
Fax: 202-357-3555
E-mail: aoainfo@aoa.hhs.gov

Eldercare Locator

Toll-free: 800-677-1116
Internet: www.eldercare.gov

The Eldercare Locator is a public service of the U.S. Administration on Aging. The Eldercare Locator connects older Americans and their caregivers with sources of information on senior services. The service links those who need assistance with state and local area agencies on aging and community-based organizations that serve older adults and their caregivers. For example, resources include Alzheimer's hotlines, adult day care and respite services, nursing home ombudsman assistance, consumer fraud, in-home care complaints, legal services, elder abuse/protective services, Medicare/Medicaid/Medigap information, tax assistance, and transportation.

National Association of Area Agencies on Aging

1730 Rhode Island Avenue, NW, Suite 1200
Washington, DC 20036
Telephone: 202-872-0888
Fax: 202-872-0057
Internet: www.n4a.org

The National Association of Area Agencies on Aging (N4A) is the umbrella organization for the 655 area agencies on aging (AAAs) and more than 230 Title VI Native American aging programs in the United States. The N4A's primary mission is to help older persons and persons with disabilities and chronic illnesses live with dignity and choices in their homes and communities for as long as possible.

National Association of Social Workers (NASW)

750 First Street, NE, Suite 700
Washington, DC 20002-4241
Toll-free: 800-638-8799
Telephone: 202-408-8600
Internet: www.socialworkers.org

The National Association of Social Workers (NASW) is the largest membership organization of professional social workers in the world. The NASW Register of Clinical Social Workers, available on the Web site under "Find a Social Worker," is a resource members of the public can use to identify social workers who are qualified by education, experience, and credentials to provide mental health services.

Resources for Children and Adolescents

Cancercare for Kids

275 Seventh Avenue, Floor 22
New York, NY 10001
Toll-free: 800-813-HOPE (800-813-4673)
E-mail: info@cancercare.org • Internet: www.cancercareforkids.org

Cancercare for Kids is an online support program for teens with a parent, sibling, or other family member who has cancer. The toll-free number is also for anyone who has cancer or has a loved one with cancer.

Cancer Really Sucks

Internet: www.cancerreallysucks.org

Cancer Really Sucks is an Internet-only resource designed for teens by teens who have loved ones facing cancer.

Kidscope

2045 Peachtree Road, Suite 150
Atlanta, GA 30309
Internet: www.kidscope.org

KidsCope is an Internet-only resource for children and families. Its mission is to help children and families understand the effects of cancer or chemotherapy on a loved one, to provide suggestions for coping, and to develop innovative programs and materials that communicate a message of hope. The site offers resources including a comic book for children about chemotherapy (Kemo Shark) and a video for kids about a mom with breast cancer.

Kids Konnected

26071 Merit Circle, Suite 103
Laguna Hills, CA 92653
Toll-free: 800-899-2866
Telephone: 949-582-5443
Email: info@kidskonnected.org
Internet: www.kidskonnected.org

Kids Konnected is a national organization that offers groups and programs for children who have a parent with cancer. They provide information, referrals to local services, a newsletter, and grief workshops.

Additional Resources

American Pain Foundation

201 N. Charles Street, Suite 710
Baltimore, MD 21201-4111
Toll-free: 888-615-PAIN (888-615-7246)
E-mail: info@painfoundation.org.
Internet: www.painfoundation.org

The American Pain Foundation is an independent nonprofit organization serving people with pain through information, advocacy, and support. Their mission is to improve the quality of life of people with pain by raising public awareness, providing practical information, promoting research, and advocating to remove barriers and increase access to effective pain management.

American College of Physicians

190 N. Independence Mall West
Philadelphia, PA 19106-1572
Toll-free: 800-523-1546
Telephone: 215-351-2400
Internet: www.acponline.org

This organization provides a free book called the *American College of Physicians Home Care Guide for Advanced Cancer* to help caregivers deal with the complex issues of caring for someone with cancer. The entire book can be viewed or downloaded from the web site at http://www.acponline.org/patients_families/end_of_life_issues/cancer/.

National Association of Hospital Hospitality Houses, Inc.

44 Merrimon Avenue, 1st Floor
Asheville, NC 28801
Toll-free: 800-542-9730
Telephone: 828-253-1188
Fax: 828-542-9730
E-mail: helpinghomes@nahhh.org • Internet: www.nahhh.com

The National Association of Hospital Hospitality Houses, Inc. (NAHHH) provides information about hospital hospitality facilities, including Ronald McDonald Houses. These facilities provide lodging and other supportive services in a home-like environment, primarily for relatives of patients seeking medical treatment outside their own community. Services vary from facility to facility and are offered at little or no cost to the guests.

American Physical Therapy Association

1111 North Fairfax Street
Alexandria, VA 22314-1488
Toll-free: 800-999-APTA (800-999-2782)
Fax: 703-684-7343
Internet: www.apta.org

The American Physical Therapy Association (APTA) is a national professional organization representing more than seventy-two thousand members. The organization represents and promotes the profession of physical therapy and strives to further the profession's role in the prevention, diagnosis, and treatment of movement dysfunctions and the enhancement of the physical health and functional abilities of members of the public. Its goal is to foster advancements in physical therapy through practice, research, and education.

International Association of Laryngectomees

925B Peachtree Street NE, Suite 316
Atlanta, GA 30309
Toll-free: 866-425-3678
Internet: www.theial.com/ial

The International Association of Laryngectomees (IAL) is a nonprofit voluntary organization composed of approximately three hundred laryngectomee member clubs. The purpose of the IAL is to assist local clubs in their efforts toward total rehabilitation of laryngectomees.

IAL programs include skills education for laryngectomees; a registry of alaryngeal (post-laryngectomy) speech instructors; the Voice Rehabilitation Institute which trains laryngectomees and therapists; and educational materials.

National Lymphedema Network

Latham Square
1611 Telegraph Avenue, Suite 111
Oakland, CA 94612-2138
Telephone: 510-208-3200
Fax: 510-208-3110
Internet: www.lymphnet.org

The National Lymphedema Network (NLN) is a nonprofit organization providing education and guidance to lymphedema patients, health care professionals, and the public by disseminating information on the prevention and management of primary and secondary lymphedema. The NLN is supported by tax-deductible donations and is a driving force behind the movement in the U.S. to standardize quality treatment for lymphedema patients nationwide. In addition, the NLN supports research into the causes and possible alternative treatments for this often incapacitating, long-neglected condition.

United Ostomy Associations of America, Inc.

P. O. Box 66
Fairview, TN 37062-0066
Toll-free: 800-826-0826
E-mail: info@uoaa.org
Internet: www.uoa.org

The United Ostomy Associations of America, Inc. (UOA) is a volunteer-based health organization dedicated to assisting people who have had or will have intestinal or urinary diversions. The UOA has more than four hundred chapters. They provide emotional support and rehabilitation programs, pre-operative and post-operative visitation programs, and networks for parents of children with ostomies. They also produce several publications, such as the *Ostomy Quarterly* magazine.

Department of Health and Human Services Medicare Hotline

7500 Security Boulevard.
Baltimore, MD 21244-1850
Toll-free: 800-MEDICARE (800-633-4227)
Internet: www.medicare.gov

The Medicare Hotline answers questions and provides literature about Medicare referral to state Medicare offices; referral to local HMOs that have contracts with Medicare; and limited information on Medicaid. The Web site includes the following services:

Medicare Compare: This interactive database includes detailed information on Medicare's health plan options. Individuals can "comparison shop" and find the plans that will work best for them.

Nursing Home Database: Detailed information on every Medicare- and Medicaid-certified nursing home is provided.

National Consumers League

1701 K Street, NW, Suite 1200
Washington, DC 20006
Telephone: 202-835-3323
Fraud Hotline: 800-876-7060
Fax: 202-835-0747

E-mail: info@nclnet.org
Internet: www.natlconsumersleague.org

The National Consumers League protects the public by providing the consumer's perspective on concerns such as medication information, privacy on the Internet, food safety, and child labor. The fraud hotline provides consumers advice about telephone solicitations and how to report possible telemarketing fraud to law enforcement agencies.

Pharmaceutical Research and Manufacturers Association of America

950 F Street NW
Washington, DC 20004
Telephone: 202-835-3400
Fax: 202-835-3414
Internet: www.phrma.org

Partnership for Prescription Assistance

Toll-free: 888-4PPA-NOW (888-477-2669)
Internet: www.pparx.org

The Partnership for Prescription Assistance helps qualifying patients without prescription drug coverage get the medicines they need through a program that is right for them. The organization provides a Directory of Prescription Drug Patient Assistance Programs that contains information about how to make a request for assistance, what prescription medicines are covered, and basic eligibility criteria.

Medicare Rights Center

520 Eighth Avenue
Northwing, 3rd Floor
New York, NY 10018
Toll-free: 800-333-4114
Telephone: 212-869-3850
Fax: 212-869-3532
E-mail: info@medicarerights.org
Internet: www.medicarerights.org

Medicare Rights Center is a national, not-for-profit, non-governmental organization that helps ensure older adults and people with disabilities get good affordable health care. It provides telephone hotline services to individuals who need answers to Medicare questions or help securing coverage and teaches people with Medicare and those who counsel them (health care providers, social service workers, family members, and others) about Medicare benefits and rights.

Patient Advocate Foundation

700 Thimble Shoals Boulevard, Suite 200
Newport News, VA 23606
Toll-free: 800-532-5274
Fax: 757-873-8999
E-mail: help@patientadvocate.org
Internet: www.patientadvocate.org

Patient Advocate Foundation (PAF) is a national nonprofit organization that provides professional case management services to Americans with chronic, life-threatening, and debilitating illnesses. PAF case managers, assisted by doctors and health care attorneys, serve as active liaisons between the patient and their insurer, employer, and/or creditors to resolve insurance, job retention, and/or debt crisis matters as they relate to their diagnoses. Patient Advocate Foundation seeks to safeguard patients through effective mediation, ensuring access to care, maintenance of employment, and preservation of their financial stability.

Assisted Living Federation of America

1650 King Street, Suite 602
Alexandria, VA 22314
Telephone: 703-894-1805
Internet: www.alfa.org

The Assisted Living Federation of America (ALFA) is an association of companies operating professionally managed assisted living communities for seniors. With more than five hundred large and small company members nationwide, ALFA serves as the voice of senior living and advocates on behalf of their members and the seniors they serve. This organization provides information about choosing an assisted living residence and publishes a consumer brochure and checklist. They also offer a searchable online directory of assisted living.

Hospice Association of America

228 Seventh Street, SE
Washington, DC 20003
Telephone: 202-546-4759
Fax: 202-547-9559
Internet: www.nahc.org/haa

The Hospice Association of America (HAA) is a trade organization with one of the largest lobbying groups for hospices in the country. It represents more than two thousand hospices and thousands of caregivers and volunteers who serve terminally ill patients and their families. The HAA distributes general information about hospice to consumers at their web site or in brochure format which can be ordered by telephone.

Hospice Foundation of America

1621 Connecticut Avenue, NW, Suite 300
Washington, DC 20009
Toll-free: 800-854-3402
Fax: (202) 638-5312
E-mail: info@hospicefoundation.org
Internet: www.hospicefoundation.org

Hospice Foundation of America (HFA) provides leadership in the development and application of hospice and its philosophy of care with the goal of enhancing the U.S. health care system and the role of hospice within it. The HFA offers a broad range of patient programs, such as information and materials on hospice care, a hospice locator service, and educational programs. Their web site has information on hospice, HFA programs and materials, and links to related sites.

Hospice Net

401 Bowling Avenue, Suite 51
Nashville, TN 37205-5124
E-mail: info@hospicenet.org
Internet: http://www.hospicenet.org

Hospice Net is an independent nonprofit organization that works exclusively through the Internet. It contains more than one hundred articles regarding end-of-life issues. Hospice nurses, social workers, bereavement counselors, and chaplains are available to answer questions via e-mail. The Web site includes information for patients and caregivers about hospice care, information about grief and loss, and a hospice locator service.

Alliance of State Pain Initiatives

University of Wisconsin School of Medicine and Public Health
1300 University Avenue
Room 4720
Madison, WI 53706
Telephone: 608-265-4013
Fax: 608-265-4014
E-mail: aspi@mailplus.wisc.edu
Internet: http://www.aacpi.wisc.edu

The Alliance of State Pain Initiatives (ASPI) is a national network of interdisciplinary, state-based organizations dedicated to transforming the culture of pain care. State Pain Initiatives are typically volunteer groups composed of nurses, physicians, pharmacists, social workers, psychologists, patient advocates, and representatives of clergy, government, and higher education who are working to improve the care of persons with pain. This network promotes the relief of cancer pain through advocacy and education by providing information for patients about pain management and developing educational, advocacy, and institutional improvement programs.

Hospice Education Institute

3 Unity Square
P. O. Box 98
Machiasport, ME 04655
Toll-free: 800-331-1620
Telephone: 207-255-8800
Fax: 207-255-8008
E-mail: info@hospiceworld.org
Internet: www.hospiceworld.org

The Hospice Education Institute provides Hospice Link, a database and directory of all hospice and palliative care organizations in the United States. It is an independent organization that provides information and education about the many facets of caring. The Institute works to inform, to educate, and to support people seeking or providing care for the dying and the bereaved, or themselves coping with far advanced illness or loss.

American Cancer Society Support Programs and Services

The American Cancer Society has free programs and services to help people with cancer and their loved ones understand cancer, manage their lives through treatment and recovery, and find the emotional support they need. For information on whether a service is available in your area, call **800-227-2345** or visit the Web site, **cancer.org**.

Cancer Survivors Network

http://csn.cancer.org
The Cancer Survivors Network (CSN) is an online community by and for people with cancer and their families. Find and connect with others through a member search, discussion boards, chat rooms, and private CSN e-mail. Create your own personal space to tell others about yourself, share photos or audio, start an online journal (blog), contribute resources, and more.

Road to Recovery℠

The Road to Recovery program provides rides to patients who have no way to get to cancer treatment.

Hope Lodge®

Each Hope Lodge offers cancer patients and their families a free, temporary place to stay when their best hope for effective treatment may be in another city. Currently, there are thirty Hope Lodge locations throughout the United States. Accommodations and eligibility requirements may vary by location, and room availability is first come, first served.

tlc

The *tlc* "magalog" is the American Cancer Society's catalog and magazine for women. It offers helpful articles and a line of products made for women with cancer. Products include wigs, hairpieces, breast forms, bras, hats, turbans, swimwear, and accessories. All proceeds from product sales go back into the American Cancer Society's programs and services for patients and survivors.

Reach to Recovery®

For more than forty years, the American Cancer Society Reach to Recovery program has helped people (female and male) cope with their breast cancer experience. Reach to Recovery matches trained volunteers with people dealing with breast cancer and its effects through face-to-face visits or by phone. Volunteers are trained to give support and up-to-date information, including literature for spouses, children, friends, and other loved ones.

Man to Man®

The Man to Man program helps men cope with prostate cancer by offering community-based education and support for patients and their family members. A core component of the program is the self-help and/or support group. Volunteers organize free monthly meetings where speakers and participants learn about and discuss information about prostate cancer, treatment, side effects, and how to cope with prostate cancer and its treatment. Programs services and activities vary depending on the location.

I Can Cope®

The American Cancer Society I Can Cope cancer education classes can help patients and their loved ones learn about cancer and how to take care of themselves.

Look Good…Feel Better

Look Good…Feel Better is a free, non-medical, brand-neutral, national public service program created to help individuals with cancer look good, improve their self-esteem, and manage their treatment and recovery with greater confidence. In a Look Good…Feel Better session, trained volunteer cosmetologists teach women how to cope with skin changes and hair loss using cosmetics and skin care products donated by the cosmetics industry.

Look Good…Feel Better for Teens

Look Good…Feel Better for Teens is a unique, free program for teenage cancer patients aged 13 to 17. It helps them cope with how cancer treatment and side effects can change the way they look. The program addresses the needs of both boys and girls.

Patient Navigator Program

The Patient Navigator program helps patients, families, and caregivers navigate the many systems needed during the cancer journey. Trained patient navigators at cancer treatment centers link those dealing with cancer to needed programs and resources. Patients can talk one-on-one with a patient navigator about their situation.

GLOSSARY

acute pain: physical discomfort that develops in a few hours or days. *See also* chronic pain.

adjuvant: aiding or supplementing; used to describe treatment administered to enhance the effects of other treatments, to treat symptoms that may increase pain, or to provide pain relief.

adjuvant therapy: treatment used in addition to the main treatment. It usually refers to hormonal therapy, chemotherapy, radiation therapy, or immunotherapy added after surgery to increase the chances of curing the disease or keeping it in check.

allogeneic bone marrow transplant: *see* bone marrow transplant (BMT).

alopecia: hair loss. Alopecia often occurs as a result of chemotherapy or radiation therapy to the head. In most cases, the hair grows back after treatment ends.

analgesic: medicine for mild pain relief, such as acetaminophen. *See also* adjuvant, nonopioid, and nonsteroidal anti-inflammatory drug (NSAID).

analog: a synthetic version of a naturally occurring substance. *See also* luteinizing hormone–releasing hormone (LHRH) analog.

androgen: any male sex hormone. The major androgen is testosterone. *See also* testosterone.

anemia: a condition in which a low red blood cell count causes a person to feel fatigued and have shortness of breath.

anesthesia: the loss of feeling or sensation as a result of medicines or gases. General anesthesia causes loss of consciousness, or "puts a person to sleep." Local or regional anesthesia numbs only a certain area of the body.

antiandrogen: a medicine that blocks the body's ability to use androgens. *See also* hormonal therapy.

antibiotics: medicines used to kill organisms that cause disease. Antibiotics may be made by living organisms or they may be created in the laboratory. Since some cancer treatments can reduce the body's ability to fight off infection, antibiotics may be used to treat or prevent these infections.

antibody: a protein produced by immune system cells and released into the blood. Antibodies defend against foreign agents, such as bacteria. These agents contain certain substances called antigens, and each antibody works against a specific antigen. See also antigen.

antiemetic: a drug that prevents or relieves nausea and vomiting, common side effects of chemotherapy.

antiestrogen: a substance or hormonal therapy (for example, the drug tamoxifen) that blocks the effects of estrogen on tumors. Antiestrogens are used to treat breast cancers that depend on estrogen for growth. *See also* hormonal therapy.

antigen: a substance that causes the body's immune system to react. This reaction often involves the production of antibodies. For example, cancer cells have certain antigens that can be found by laboratory tests; they are important in cancer diagnosis and in watching response to treatment. *See also* antibody.

anxiety: a mental state of uncertainty, fear, and nervousness resulting from a real or perceived threatening event or situation. Prolonged or severe anxiety can result in impaired day-to-day functioning. People with cancer and caregivers commonly experience anxiety and fear.

apheresis: a simplified process for harvesting peripheral stem cells for transplantation. Also called leukapheresis.

aromatase inhibitor: a drug that stops estrogen production.

autologous bone marrow transplant: *see* bone marrow transplant (BMT).

benign: not cancerous; not malignant.

biological therapy: a type of cancer treatment that boosts the body's immune system to fight against cancer or lessens the side effects of some cancer treatments. Interferon is one example. Also called biological response modifier therapy, biotherapy, or immunotherapy.

biologic response modifier (BRM): naturally occurring substance in the body that changes the interaction between the body's immune defenses and cancer, improving the body's ability to fight the disease.

biopsy: the removal of a sample of tissue to see whether cancer cells are present. *See also* core needle biopsy, excisional biopsy, fine needle aspiration (FNA), incisional biopsy, and needle biopsy.

blood count: a count of the number of red blood cells and white blood cells in a given sample of blood.

bone marrow: the soft tissue in the hollow of flat bones of the body that produces new blood cells.

bone marrow transplant (BMT): a complex treatment used when cancer is advanced or has recurred or used as the main treatment in some types of leukemia or lymphoma. An *autologous BMT* uses bone marrow from the person with cancer. An *allogeneic BMT* uses marrow from a donor whose tissue type closely matches that of the person getting the treatment. A *syngeneic BMT* occurs when the donor is an identical twin.

brachytherapy: internal radiation treatment given by placing radioactive material directly into the tumor or close to it. Also called interstitial radiation therapy or seed implantation. *See also* internal radiation, interstitial radiation therapy.

breakthrough pain: pain that causes discomfort between scheduled times for giving pain medicine.

cachexia: a profound state of general poor health and malnutrition (poor dietary intake).

cancer: a group of diseases that causes cells in the body to change and grow out of control. Most types of cancer cells form a lump or mass called a tumor. Cells from the tumor can break away and travel to other parts of the body, where they can continue to grow. This spreading process is called metastasis. *See also* neoplasm.

caregiver: one who provides direct care, helping maintain or restore health and supporting the dignity, independence, and quality of life of the person under care.

catheter: a thin, flexible tube through which fluids enter or leave the body (for example, a tube to drain urine). A central venous catheter is one that is placed in a vein in the body and remains there as long as it is needed. *See also* intra-arterial catheter, intracavitary catheter, intrathecal catheter, peripherally inserted central catheter (PICC).

chemotherapy: treatment with medicines to destroy cancer cells. Chemotherapy is often used with surgery or radiation to treat cancer when the cancer has spread, when it has come back (recurred), or when there is a strong chance that it could recur. *See also* systemic therapy.

chronic pain: ongoing physical discomfort that lasts three months or more. *See also* acute pain.

clinical trials: research studies to test new medicines or other treatments to compare current standard treatments with others that may be better.

colostomy: an opening in the abdomen for getting rid of body waste (feces). A colostomy is sometimes needed after surgery for cancer of the rectum.

conditioning: treatment with high-dose chemotherapy with or without radiation therapy that is usually used before stem cell transplantation.

constipation: a condition that occurs when bowel movements happen less often than usual and when stools are hard or difficult to move. Constipation can be caused by medicines used to treat cancer, such as narcotics; emotional stress; changes in diet; and decreased activity.

core needle biopsy: the removal of a cylindrical sample of tissue from a tumor for microscopic analysis using a relatively thick needle.

corticosteroid: any of a number of steroid substances obtained from the cortex of the adrenal glands. Used in hormonal therapy or to reduce persistent nausea, corticosteroids are sometimes called steroids. *See also* hormonal therapy.

cryosurgery: a surgical technique that uses liquid nitrogen spray or a very cold probe to freeze and kill abnormal cells. Also called cryoablation.

curative surgery: removal of a tumor when cancer appears to be localized and there is hope of removing all of the cancerous tissue.

cyclooxygenase-2 inhibitor: a type of nonsteroidal anti-inflammatory drug that is used as a pain reliever but has been linked to increased cardiovascular problems. Relief occurs because the drug blocks prostaglandins that have been shown to promote arthritis pain and swelling. Also called cox-2 inhibitor and selective cyclooxygenase inhibitor.

depression: a psychiatric disorder characterized by a lack of concentration, insomnia or over-sleeping, loss of appetite, feelings of extreme sadness, guilt, helplessness and hopelessness, and thoughts of death. Some cancer medicines can cause symptoms of depression. Clinical depression is also referred to as major depression.

diagnostic surgery: surgery used to obtain a tissue sample for laboratory testing to confirm a diagnosis and identify the specific cancer.

diarrhea: liquid stools that result from frequent bowel movements and that feel more urgent than normal stools.

diethylstilbestrol (DES): a synthetic form of estrogen. At one time, DES was the main form of hormonal therapy for men with prostate cancer. *See also* hormonal therapy.

dry orgasm: in a man, the feeling of an orgasm without ejaculation.

edema: buildup of fluid in the tissues, causing swelling. Edema of the arm or leg can occur after surgery or radiation. *See also* lymphedema.

electrosurgery: a surgical procedure that involves the use of high-frequency electrical current to destroy cells.

emesis: vomiting.

endoscopy: inspection of body organs or cavities using a flexible, lighted tube called an endoscope.

enema: the injection of liquid, such as mineral oil, chemically treated water, or soap suds, into the rectum (lower bowel) for cleansing, for stimulating a bowel movement, or for other therapeutic or diagnostic purposes; a stool softener for relief of constipation.

engraftment: the beginning of the growth of transplanted stem cells in a recipient's bone marrow.

enterostomal therapist: a health professional, often a nurse, who teaches people how to care for ostomies (surgically created openings, such as colostomies) and other wounds.

estrogen: a female sex hormone produced primarily by the ovaries and in smaller amounts by the adrenal cortex. *See also* hormone replacement therapy, hormonal therapy.

excisional biopsy: a type of diagnostic surgery in which a surgeon removes an entire tumor for testing.

external radiation: radiation focused from a source outside the body on an area affected by the cancer. It is much like getting a diagnostic x-ray, but exposures are repeated and each lasts longer than an x-ray.

feces: human solid waste matter, bowel movement, or stool.

fiber: dietary fiber includes a wide variety of plant carbohydrates that are not digested by humans. Fibers are classified as soluble (for example, oat bran) and insoluble (for example, wheat bran). Good sources of fiber are beans, vegetables, whole grains, and fruits.

fibrosis: formation of scarlike (fibrous) tissue. This can occur anywhere in the body.

fine needle aspiration (FNA): in this procedure, a thin needle is used to withdraw (aspirate) sample cells, fluid, or other matter for examination under a microscope. *See* biopsy and needle biopsy.

gastrointestinal (GI) tract: the digestive (or intestinal) tract. It consists of those organs and structures that process and prepare food to be used for energy, including the stomach, small intestine, and large intestine.

GI tube: a temporary or permanent tube inserted into an opening that goes directly into the gastrointestinal (GI) tract. If a person cannot swallow food, GI tubes are sometimes used to put a thick nutritious fluid into the stomach.

hematoma: a collection of blood outside a blood vessel caused by a leak or an injury.

home health nurse: a nursing professional who gives medications in the home, teaches patients how to care for themselves, and assesses their condition to see if further medical attention is needed.

hormonal therapy: treatment with hormones, with medicines that interfere with hormone production or hormone action, or the surgical removal of hormone-producing glands. Hormonal therapy may kill cancer cells or slow their growth. Also called hormone therapy. *See also* antiandrogen, antiestrogen, aromatase inhibitor, corticosteroid, diethylstilbestrol (DES), estrogen, intermittent hormonal therapy, luteinizing hormone–releasing hormone (LHRH) analog, progestin, and total androgen blockade.

hormone: a chemical substance released into the body by the endocrine glands, such as the thyroid gland, adrenal gland, or ovaries. Hormones travel through the bloodstream and set in motion various body functions. Testosterone and estrogen are examples of male and female hormones, respectively. *See also* androgen, corticosteroid, estrogen, luteinizing hormone-releasing hormone (LHRH), progestin, and testosterone.

hormone replacement therapy: in women, the use of estrogen and progesterone from an outside source after the body has stopped making them because of natural or induced menopause.

hospice: a special kind of care for people in the final phase of illness, their families, and caregivers; also a place where such care is given. The care may take place in the person's home or in a homelike facility.

hyperalimentation: a method of giving nutrition other than as food, often intravenously. *See also* GI tube.

ileostomy: an operation in which the end of the small intestine, the ileum, is brought out through an opening in the abdomen. The contents of the intestine (unformed stool) are expelled through this opening into a bag called an appliance. *See also* ostomy.

immune system: the complex system by which the body resists infection by microbes, such as bacteria or viruses, and rejects transplanted tissues or organs. The immune system may also help the body fight some cancers. *See also* lymphatic system.

immunotherapy: treatment that promotes or supports the immune system's response to a disease such as cancer.

impotence: not being able to have or keep an erection of the penis.

incision: a cut made in the skin with a knife.

incisional biopsy: a type of diagnostic surgery in which the surgeon removes for testing a small part of tissue suspected of being cancerous.

incontinence: partial or complete loss of urinary control.

informed consent: agreement to participate in a study and/or to undergo treatment after understanding a course of treatment, including the risks, benefits, and possible alternatives, usually described in a legal document; the process by which people agree to treatment.

infusion: introduction of a solution into the body through a vein for therapeutic purposes, usually lasting thirty minutes or more.

intensity-modulated radiation therapy: a type of radiotherapy that, better than conventional therapy, prevents or moderates exposure to normal tissues, increases radiation to the tumor, and generally administers radiation with more precision by conforming to the tumor's shape.

intermittent hormonal therapy: a type of prostate cancer treatment in which hormonal medicines are stopped after a man's blood prostate-specific antigen (PSA) level drops to a very low level and remains stable for a while. If the PSA level begins to rise, the medicines are started again. *See also* hormonal therapy.

internal radiation: treatment involving implantation of a radioactive substance. *See also* brachytherapy, interstitial radiation therapy.

interstitial radiation therapy: a type of internal radiation (or brachytherapy) treatment in which a radioactive implant is placed directly into the tissue (not in a body cavity).

intraarterial catheter: a catheter that delivers fluids directly into an artery to treat a specific part of the body.

intracavitary catheter: a catheter that is placed in the abdomen, pelvis, or chest.

intrathecal catheter: a catheter that delivers fluids into the spinal fluid.

intravenous (IV): a method of supplying fluids and medications using a needle inserted in a vein.

intravenous (IV) catheter: *see* catheter.

insomnia: the inability to sleep. In the person with cancer, insomnia can occur as a result of pain.

investigational: under study; often used to describe medicines used in clinical trials.

IV push: medicines delivered through a thin needle inserted into a vein, given over a few minutes. *See also* infusion.

laparoscopy: examination of the abdominal cavity with a long, slender tube (a laparoscope) that allows doctors to see and photograph what they see. The tube is inserted into the abdomen through a very small incision; similar to endoscopy.

laparotomy: a surgical procedure that opens the abdominal wall. May include examination and biopsy of tissue from the abdominal cavity with a laparoscope. This examination may be done when there is uncertainty about a suspicious area that cannot be diagnosed by less intrusive tests.

laryngectomy: surgery to remove the voice box (larynx), usually because of cancer.

laser surgery: a type of surgery using laser (light amplification by stimulated emission of radiation) light. Laser light is a highly focused, powerful beam of light energy used in medicine for precise and relatively noninvasive surgical work.

laxative: a food or drug that stimulates the bowels to move waste products out of the body. For the person with cancer, a laxative may ease constipation caused by pain medicines.

leukapheresis: *see* apheresis.

luteinizing hormone–releasing hormone (LHRH): a hormone produced by the hypothalamus, a tiny gland in the brain, which affects levels of luteinizing hormone in the body and therefore affects testosterone levels.

luteinizing hormone–releasing hormone (LHRH) analog: manufactured hormone, chemically similar to luteinizing hormone–releasing hormone. It blocks the production of the male hormone testosterone and is sometimes used as a treatment for prostate cancer. *See also* hormonal therapy, luteinizing hormone–releasing hormone (LHRH).

lymphatic system: the tissues and organs (including lymph nodes, spleen, thymus, and bone marrow) that produce and store lymphocytes (cells that fight infection) and the channels that carry the lymph fluid. The entire lymphatic system is an important part of the body's immune system. Invasive cancers sometimes penetrate the lymphatic vessels and spread (metastasize) to lymph nodes. *See also* immune system.

lymphedema: a complication in which excess fluid collects in the arms or legs. This often happens after the lymph nodes and vessels are removed during surgery, after injury by radiation, or when a tumor interferes with normal drainage of the fluid (such as after breast cancer treatments). This condition can be persistent but not painful. *See also* edema.

lymph nodes: small bean-shaped collections of immune system tissue, such as lymphocytes, found along lymphatic vessels. They remove cell waste and fluids from lymph. They help fight infections and also have a role in fighting cancer.

manic depression: a mental illness characterized by alternating episodes of mania (changing ideas, exaggerated sexuality, excessive happiness or irritability, and decreased sleep) and depression. Also called bipolar illness or manic-depressive illness. *See also* depression.

metastasis: the spread of cancer cells to distant areas of the body through the lymph system or bloodstream.

mucositis: inflammation of the mucous membranes of the digestive tract, particularly those of the mouth. Used interchangeably with stomatitis.

needle biopsy: needle-facilitated removal of fluid, cells, or tissue for examination under a microscope. There are two types: fine needle aspiration (FNA) and core biopsy.

neoadjuvant therapy: a systemic therapy, such as chemotherapy or hormonal therapy, given before surgery or radiation. This type of therapy can shrink some tumors so that they are easier to remove.

neoplasm: an abnormal growth (tumor) that starts from a single altered cell. A neoplasm may be benign or malignant. Cancer is a malignant neoplasm. *See* also tumor.

neuropathic pain: physical discomfort, often described as burning or shooting, that originates in the nerves.

nonopioid: mild to moderate pain reliever, such as acetaminophen, aspirin, and ibuprofen. Many nonopioids are over-the-counter medicines (do not require a prescription). *See also* analgesic, nonsteroidal anti-inflammatory drug (NSAID).

nonsteroidal anti-inflammatory drug (NSAID): a mild pain reliever. Examples include aspirin and ibuprofen. Check with your doctor before using these medicines. NSAIDs can slow blood clotting, especially if you are on chemotherapy. *See also* analgesic, nonopioid.

opioid: prescription narcotic medicine used to relieve pain. Some examples include codeine, morphine, and fentanyl.

ostomy: a general term meaning an opening, especially one made by surgery. An ostomy is not a disease; rather, it is a change in anatomy that may be necessary as a result of a disease or condition. Not all ostomies are permanent. *See also* colostomy, ileostomy, stoma, tracheostomy, and urostomy.

palliative treatment: treatment that relieves symptoms, such as pain, but is not designed to cure the disease. Its main purpose is to improve the person's quality of life. *Palliative surgery* is surgery performed to treat complications of advanced disease and to correct a condition that is causing discomfort or disability.

peripheral blood stem cell transplantation (PBSCT): stem cells used for transplantation are usually obtained from the peripheral blood (bloodstream) by a procedure called *apheresis* (also called *leukapheresis*). Apheresis is undergone and the cells stored before the patient is treated with large doses of chemotherapy or radiation. After treatment, the patient receives a transplant of the stem cells to restore the blood-producing bone marrow stem cells. There are three main types of SCTs—allogeneic, autologous, and syngeneic. *See also* bone marrow transplant (BMT).

peripherally inserted central catheter (PICC): a type of catheter that allows continuous access to a large arm vein for several weeks.

platelet: a specific blood cell that plugs holes in blood vessels after an injury. Chemotherapy can cause a drop in the platelet count, a condition called *thrombocytopenia*, that carries a risk of excessive bleeding.

premalignant: changes in cells that may, but do not always, become cancer. Also called precancerous.

preventive surgery: surgery performed to remove a growth that is not yet malignant (cancerous) but is likely to become malignant if left untreated. Sometimes also called prophylactic surgery.

primary site or tumor: the place where cancer begins. Primary cancer is usually named after the organ in which it starts.

prn: as the situation demands; as needed. Used in writing prescriptions or referring to taking medicines. From the Latin *pro re nata*, or "for the thing born."

progesterone: a female sex hormone released by the ovaries during every menstrual cycle to prepare the uterus for pregnancy and the breasts for milk production (lactation).

progestin: a hormone produced in the ovaries; a hormone used in treatment for advanced breast cancer after other hormone treatments have been tried. *See also* hormonal therapy.

prognosis: a prediction of the course of disease; the outlook for the cure of the person who is ill.

prosthesis: an artificial form, such as a breast or leg prosthesis, that replaces a part of the body.

protocol: a formalized outline or plan describing what treatments a patient will receive and exactly when each should be given. *See also* regimen.

proton therapy: a type of radiation therapy that uses particle beams and is known for its ability to spare normal tissues. Advantages include improved control of the therapeutic beam, the protons, which can be made to conform to the shape of the tumor and to stop before penetrating into normal tissues beyond the tumor.

radiation therapy: treatment with radiation (high-energy particles or waves, such as x-rays, gamma rays, electrons, and protons) to destroy cancer cells. This type of treatment may be used to reduce the size of a cancer before surgery; to destroy any remaining cancer cells after surgery; or, in some cases, as the main treatment. Also called irradiation, radiotherapy, and x-ray therapy. *See also* external radiation, internal radiation.

rectum: the lower part of the large intestine leading to the anus.

recurrence: cancer that has come back after treatment appeared to have removed evidence of the disease.

regimen: a strict, regulated plan (such as diet, exercise, or other activity) designed to reach certain goals. In cancer treatment, a regimen is a plan to treat cancer. *See also* protocol.

rehabilitation: activities to help a person adjust, heal, and return to a full, productive life after injury or illness. This may involve physical restoration (such as the use of prostheses, exercises, and physical therapy), counseling, and emotional support.

remission: complete or partial disappearance of the signs and symptoms of cancer in response to treatment; the period during which a disease is under control. A remission may not be a cure.

restorative surgery: surgery used to restore a person's appearance or restore the function of an organ or body part. Also called reconstructive surgery.

risk factor: anything that increases a person's chance of getting a disease such as cancer.

secondary tumor: a tumor that forms as a result of the spread (metastasis) of cancer from the place where it started.

side effects: unintended and usually undesirable effects of treatment, such as hair loss or fatigue.

simulation: the process a radiation therapist uses to identify where to direct radiation.

somatic pain: physical discomfort, including aching or throbbing, that arises from bone, joint, muscle, or skin.

staging: the process of finding out whether cancer has spread and if so, how far. There is more than one system for staging cancer.

staging surgery: surgery performed to determine how far disease has spread.

stem cells: immature cells that eventually develop into circulating blood cells. Stem cells mostly live in the bone marrow, where they produce blood cells. They have the ability to change into different types of blood cells needed by the body.

steroid: *see* corticosteroid.

stoma: an opening, especially an opening made by surgery to allow elimination of body waste. *See also* ostomy.

stomatitis: inflammation or ulcers of the mouth area. This condition can be a side effect of some chemotherapies. Used interchangeably with mucositis.

subcutaneous: located or placed just beneath the skin.

supportive surgery: surgery used to help with other types of treatment, such as the delivery of pain medicine or chemotherapy (via a peripherally inserted central catheter).

surgery: the treatment of disease, injury, or disfigurement with an operation. Surgery is the oldest form of treatment for cancer and offers the greatest chance for cure. *See also* diagnostic surgery, laser surgery, palliative treatment, preventive surgery, restorative surgery, staging surgery, supportive surgery.

syngeneic bone marrow transplant: *see* bone marrow transplant (BMT).

systemic therapy: treatment (for example, chemotherapy) that reaches and affects cells throughout the body. *See also* neoadjuvant therapy.

testosterone: a male sex hormone, made primarily in the testes. In men with prostate cancer, it can also encourage growth of the tumor.

thrombocytopenia: a condition characterized by a low level of platelets in the blood; it can be a side effect of chemotherapy.

thrush: a treatable infection of the mouth or esophagus; a temporary side effect of chemotherapy or radiation therapy to the throat or chest.

total androgen blockade: a treatment that combines antiandrogen and luteinizing hormone–releasing hormone (LHRH) analog therapy with orchiectomy (removal of the testicles) to block the body's ability to produce and use androgens. Also called combination hormone therapy, combined androgen blockade (CAB), total androgen ablation, total androgen blockade, or total hormonal ablation. *See also* antiandrogen, hormonal therapy, luteinizing hormone–releasing hormone (LHRH) analog.

tracheostomy: surgery to create an opening in the trachea (windpipe) through the neck.

transdermal skin patch: a method of drug delivery in which a patch is placed on the body and delivers medicine through the skin for up to seventy-two hours.

transmucosal administration: a method of drug delivery in which medicine is absorbed through the lining of the mouth (by putting the medicine inside the cheek or between the cheek and gums). This method is usually used when a patient cannot ingest tablets or liquid because of difficulty swallowing.

tumor: an abnormal lump or mass of tissue. Tumors can be benign (not cancerous) or malignant (cancerous). *See also* neoplasm.

urostomy: surgery to divert urine through a new passage and then through an opening in the abdomen. In a continent urostomy, the urine is stored inside the body and drained a few times a day through a tube placed into an opening called a *stoma.*

venipuncture: the puncture of a vein, usually to draw blood or to inject a substance. *See also* intravenous (IV).

visceral pain: physical discomfort, often described as cramping, that arises from organs, including the stomach or liver.

x-rays: one form of radiation that can be used at low levels to produce an image of the body on film or at high levels to destroy cancer cells. *See also* radiation therapy.

INDEX

for teens, 24
for transportation services, 47
warning about, xvii
weight gain, avoiding, 224
weight loss
adjusting medicine dosage, 212
at end of life, 249

rapid, 163, 164
slowing, 169–171
white blood cell count, low, 117, 121, 123, 290–291
wigs, 193–194, 195
Wong-Baker FACES Pain Rating Scale, 126–127
World Health Organization pain relief approach, 131

About the Editors

Julia A. Bucher, RN, PhD, is an associate professor in the Department of Nursing at York College of Pennsylvania, where she teaches Community Health Nursing. Her previous experience includes caring for people with cancer at home and helping their families as a cancer clinical nurse specialist. She has designed and evaluated several types of supportive community services to help people with cancer and their families cope. Dr. Bucher uses a problem-solving approach to teach students and families how to deal with problems using a focused, step-by-step approach. She received her PhD in community systems planning and development from Penn State in 1992 and has been affiliated with the American Cancer Society for several decades as a volunteer, statewide planner, and data manager. She is dedicated to making life easier for those facing the cancer challenge.

Peter S. Houts, PhD, is a retired professor of behavioral science at Penn State University College of Medicine. A social psychologist, Dr. Houts has conducted research for more than twenty-five years on how cancer patients cope with their illness. He has developed and evaluated innovative interventions to help cancer patients and their family caregivers cope with illness. He has also directed surveys focusing on the problems and unmet needs of people dealing with a cancer diagnosis. Dr. Houts was a co-developer of the psychoeducational COPE Model, which is widely used in applying problem-solving techniques to cope with illness. He continues to mentor colleagues and act as a consultant on research dealing with applying problem-solving education and counseling to health care. Dr. Houts is coauthor of numerous publications on caring for cancer patients and helping those dealing with cancer to cope with it effectively.

Terri Ades, DNP, FNP-BC, AOCN, is director of Cancer Information for the American Cancer Society National Home Office in Atlanta. In this position, she oversees the development and maintenance of the Society's cancer information that is available through the Society's Web site, toll-free call center, patient education/consumer awareness materials, and translations. Dr. Ades is an oncology clinician and expert in health literacy. She is certified as an advanced practice oncology nurse and family nurse practitioner. She is an Adjunct Faculty member of Emory University Nell Hodgson Woodruff School of Nursing and the Winship Cancer Institute of Emory Healthcare where she continues in clinical practice in the Hematology Outpatient Clinic at Grady.

Other Books Published by the American Cancer Society

Available everywhere books are sold and online at **www.cancer.org/bookstore**

TOOLS FOR THE HEALTH CONSCIOUS

American Cancer Society's Healthy Eating Cookbook, Third Edition
Celebrate! Healthy Entertaining for Any Occasion
Good for You! Reducing Your Risk of Developing Cancer
The Great American Eat-Right Cookbook
Kicking Butts: Quit Smoking and Take Charge of Your Health, Second Edition

INFORMATION FOR PEOPLE WITH CANCER

American Cancer Society Complete Guide to Complementary and Alternative Cancer Therapies, Second Edition
American Cancer Society Complete Guide to Nutrition for Cancer Survivors, Second Edition
American Cancer Society's Guide to Pain Control, Revised Edition
Lymphedema: Understanding and Managing Lymphedema After Cancer Treatment
What to Eat During Cancer Treatment: 100 Great-Tasting, Family-Friendly Recipes to Help You Cope

SUPPORT FOR FAMILIES AND CAREGIVERS

Cancer Caregiving A to Z: An At-Home Guide for Patients and Families
The Survivorship Net: A Parable for the Family, Friends, and Caregivers of People with Cancer
What Helped Get Me Through: Cancer Survivors Share Wisdom and Hope

BOOKS FOR CHILDREN

Because... Someone I Love Has Cancer
Get Better! Communication Cards for Kids & Adults
Healthy Me: A Read-Along Coloring & Activity Book
Imagine What's Possible: Using the Power of Your Mind to Take Control of Your Life During Cancer
Kids' First Cookbook: Delicious-Nutritious Treats to Make Yourself!
Let My Colors Out
The Long and the Short of It: A Tale About Hair
Mom and the Polka-Dot Boo-Boo
Nana, What's Cancer?
No Thanks, but I'd Love to Dance: Choosing to Live Smoke Free

Our Dad Is Getting Better

Our Mom Has Cancer (available in hardcover and paperback)

Our Mom Is Getting Better

What's Up with Bridget's Mom? Medikidz Explain Breast Cancer (also available in Spanish)

What's Up with Jo? Medikidz Explain Brain Tumors

What's Up with Lyndon? Medikidz Explain Osteosarcoma

What's Up with Richard? Medikidz Explain Leukemia (also available in Spanish)

What's Up with Tiffany's Dad? Medikidz Explain Melanoma

Visit **cancer.org/bookstore** for a full listing of books published by the American Cancer Society.